MEDICO-LEGAL ESSENTIALS

Clinical Responsibility

MEDICO-LEGAL ESSENTIALS

Clinical Responsibility

JANE LYNCH
LLB (Hons), Legal Dip, Solicitor, FRSM

Forewords by

TIM PETTIS
Strategic Emergency Planning Manager
Acting Head of Emergency Preparedness Training
Emergency Response Department
Centre for Emergency Preparedness and Response
Health Protection Agency

and

AHMED SHOKA
Consultant Psychiatrist & Lead Clinician
North Essex Partnership Foundation Trust

Radcliffe Publishing
Oxford • New York

Radcliffe Publishing Ltd
18 Marcham Road
Abingdon
Oxon OX14 1AA
United Kingdom

www.radcliffe-oxford.com
Electronic catalogue and worldwide online ordering facility.

British Library Cataloguing in Publication Data

A catalogue record for this book is available from the British Library.

ISBN-13: 978 184619 223 4

The paper used for the text pages of this book is FSC certified. FSC (The Forest Stewardship Council) is an international network to promote responsible management of the world's forests.

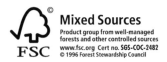

Mixed Sources
Product group from well-managed forests and other controlled sources
www.fsc.org Cert no. SGS-COC-2482
© 1996 Forest Stewardship Council

Typeset by Pindar New Zealand, Auckland, New Zealand
Printed and bound by TJI Digital, Padstow, Cornwall, UK

Contents

Foreword

This book is fascinating!

As a registered healthcare professional myself I was intrigued as I thought, before reading this book, that I was aware of the basic clinical responsibilities that I and other health professionals have to follow. How wrong I was!

This book, written by Jane Lynch (a recognised legal specialist in healthcare matters) explains very clearly and precisely – and in plain English – the processes and procedures specifically for healthcare professionals.

Each chapter is well set out with examples, scenarios and real case histories describing when things have gone wrong. The necessary actions and vital information needed to prevent those situations from arising in the first place have been a real eye opener.

I wholeheartedly recommend this book, which will become a valuable set text for all healthcare professionals. You should always keep this book to hand as a superb source for reference, alongside the other reference material you use daily in discharging your healthcare duties.

Tim Pettis
MSc BA(Hons) Cert Ed FCODP FIEM FFHEPIEM FICDDS MEPS MIAEM
Strategic Emergency Planning Manager
Acting Head of Emergency Preparedness Training
Emergency Response Department
Centre for Emergency Preparedness and Response
Health Protection Agency
Porton Down, Wiltshire
April 2009

Foreword

The relationship between medicine and law has always been interesting.

This concept has recently moved into another dimension for both health-care workers and law personnel. If it was thought to be a mere advantage for a healthcare worker to grasp some basic concepts of the medical law, it has now become a real necessity for them to understand how the medical law works, and what the wider and specific implication of the law is in daily routine clinical work.

This book is very well written and is simple to follow on a dry subject such as the law. Throughout, its content and the examples given are well structured and enlightening. It is very clear, concise and also practical.

On a personal note, I had the privilege to enjoy reading the book and learning from its content. Certainly it is a positive step in the right direction to fill the gap between medicine and law. I would recommend reading this book for all healthcare workers – whatever their level or expertise may be.

Dr Ahmed Shoka
Consultant Psychiatrist & Lead Clinician
North Essex Partnership Foundation Trust
April 2009

Preface

For health professionals the threat of the law has become a daily concern. Whilst accountability is a word that is widely used amongst health professionals they often do not sit back and think, 'what does accountability really mean?' This book explains the issues of accountability and responsibilities of the health professional in clear language using case studies and examples to illustrate the points. Its intention is not to teach the health professional how to be an amateur lawyer, but to explain the real issues of legal and professional accountability of the health professional. Foremost, it will put the legal issues into perspective so that the health professional does not constantly live in fear of being sued.

Accountability is often not wholly appreciated by the health professional. They will often assume that if they have been told to do something by their boss, or they were following a protocol, that they cannot be held personally accountable if something goes wrong and the patient suffers harm as a result. This approach is not supported in law and the health professional would indeed be personally accountable in the circumstances.

There are many pressures and demands placed on health professionals in this current climate – lack of funding and reduced staffing levels to name a few. For the health professional, can they really be held liable when a patient is harmed because of lack of training or lack of resources which are outside their control? Health professionals will say 'surely the court will have some sympathy for me because of the pressure I was under due to lack of staff', but this is not so.

The law is applied strictly. The court will have no sympathy for a health professional who says 'I am sorry the patient died, but I did not have time to write the records.'

As a lawyer it is very easy to say 'this is the law'. In practice I have every sympathy for the health professional amidst the demands and pressures and inherent conflicts they face on a daily basis. However, the legal framework exists and cannot be ignored. It is important that health professionals understand their legal and professional obligations.

Sometimes there is an unhealthy balance on the part of both patient and the Trust or the employer of the understanding of the legal issues of accountability. A patient will often demand a particular course of treatment or medication and if they do not get what they want they will threaten to sue. The Trust will sometimes give the patient what they want to avoid being sued. However, in order for a patient to sue there are several legal hurdles that must be overcome. A legal claim cannot be determined simply because there has been an adverse outcome. This is widely misunderstood by both patients and health professionals. As much as the Trusts would like to, they do not have infinite resources to give all patients the best and most expensive medication and treatment.

It is important for the health professional to understand the complexities of accountability, when and how the legal processes interact and the implications for the health professional.

It is not possible for me to fix the NHS and it is not my intention in this book to teach health professionals how to become amateur lawyers. This book looks at the areas of accountability, the legal process, what constitutes a legal claim brought by the patient, the duty of care and how it is measured. It will assist and guide the health professional in understanding their legal and professional obligations and implications for managing risk.

The law is constantly changing and evolving so whilst information contained in this book is current at the time of writing, it may change over time. The health professional has an obligation to keep abreast of the law that affects them as they are responsible for ensuring their knowledge is up to date. Remember, ignorance of the law is no defence.

The examples used are drawn from situations faced by health professionals and real cases. The basic principles should be taken and applied to the health professional's own situations. Throughout the book many questions will be posed for the reader to consider. This is to raise awareness of the issues and to get the reader thinking. There are useful examples and checklists.

With regard to terminology, throughout the text for ease of reference, the word 'health professional' is used to include doctors, nurses, allied health professionals and others involved in healthcare.

The word 'patient' is used to include the patient or the client. The words 'he' and 'she' are used randomly throughout. This is not intended to be derogatory or sexist, but simply provides easier reading.

I am very grateful to all those who contributed to this book. I am grateful to Tim Pettis and Dr Shoka for painstakingly reading the drafts and writing the Forewords to the book. To my mother, my daughter Kate for their proof reading, enthusiasm, encouragement, support and patience during my writing of this book and to whom this book is dedicated.

Jane Lynch
April 2009

About the author

Jane Lynch is a practising lawyer specialising in clinical negligence. She was a partner at a City of London firm specialising in clinical negligence. She is on The Law Society's specialist clinical negligence panel and is recognised as one of the leading practitioners in England and Wales.

She is a fellow of the Royal Society of Medicine. Jane is also a legal trainer for the health sector and is involved in training over 250 NHS Trusts, the private health sector, local authorities, public bodies, professional bodies and the MOD.

Jane is a regular speaker at international conferences and also lectures at several universities on the masters degree courses. She has had several papers and articles published, is well known in the health sector and is very highly regarded in her field.

She is a founding director of the Practical Legal Training Agency (www. plta.co.uk), which specialises in legal training for non-lawyers.

CHAPTER 1

Introduction

Over the recent past the ethos in healthcare has changed. Gone are the days when a doctor was put on a pedestal and not to be challenged, when it was routine to simply say to a patient 'nice to see you, fix you tomorrow', when health records were marked 'not to be handled by the patient'!

Now, of course, we live in a very different world. Patients are much more aware of their rights. Access to the internet has opened a huge arena for exchange of information, allowing patients to be more informed.

There is the law relating to consent. The health professional has an obligation to obtain consent of the patient before they can treat them. If they fail to comply with the rules of consent, they are in danger of commit-ting a criminal offence.

Patients now have a legal right to access to their records and indeed we now have patient-held records. Health professionals have a legal obligation to keep patient information confidential. This causes practical problems for the health professional when sharing information. If they do not comply with the issues of confidentiality they will be accountable.

For health professionals this means that the law has become part of their role and is now an everyday concern. The complexities of the law do not make this an easy task for them. In a healthcare setting, it leaves the health professionals vulnerable. In practice, they go about their daily routines, making decisions about patient care, planning and treatment and it is hoped that the right decisions are made and that the employer will stand by them and courts will uphold their decisions.

Health professionals have concerns about who is responsible when a patient suffers harm. Can a health professional be held accountable where they have no control over resources or they are ignorant through lack of training?

Health professionals are often heard in the witness box saying, 'Staff were under pressure, but I meant well. I acted in good faith.'

Of course health professionals do not intend to cause harm; they may have no control over resources; they may be ignorant of procedures through lack of training. But this does not exonerate health professionals from their responsibility. So when something goes awry they are accountable.

It is important for health professionals not only to be aware of their legal and professional obligations, but also to put them into perspective, to get the balance right. Often health professionals have an unhealthy fear of the law, causing unnecessary anxiety. This approach is balanced by an unrealistic view that it will never happen to them; that someone else or something else is responsible, 'but not me'. Often a defensive approach is adopted. 'I don't have the time'; 'it's because of financial constraints'; 'it's my manager's responsibility'; or 'it's the consultant's responsibility'. The health professional cannot simply pass responsibility onto someone else. They will be accountable for their actions.

My intention in writing this book is not to alarm the health professional unduly, but to impart the information realistically in a way that a balance may be struck and so remove the spectre of the court.

We shall look at how the court process works: the different types of court processes, the difference between the civil and criminal process and how a health professional might become involved in those court processes.

We will look at a legal claim: how a patient may sue for clinical negligence; what the patient needs to prove in order for any claim to succeed; what the duty of care is, how the duty of care is measured, what constitutes a breach of duty of care and to whom is the duty of care owed. What are the consequences for the health professional when a patient sues for clinical negligence? Who pays the compensation?

Then there are the professional implications: when and how the health professional is accountable to the professional bodies and what the consequences are.

There are issues in the course of employment: governance and risk management, a breach of contract of employment, accountability for team decisions, following orders, following guidelines and protocols, waiting lists, prescribing, lack of resources and poor record-keeping, amongst other things.

It is important that the health professional understands the separate areas of accountability as this is the underlying premise of their responsibility and all that flows from it.

THE HIGH COST OF LITIGATION

The NHS litigation authority (NHSLA) in their annual report (November 2008) stated that as of March 2008, it estimated that it had potential liabilities of £11.9 **billion** relating to clinical negligence claims.[1] This staggering figure does not include the cost of staff and management time in dealing with these complaints or the additional cost of bed space. So the true cost is far higher. This figure represents something in the region of 10% of the annual budget. If you compare this with the prescription budget, which is around 8%, you can see how much litigation is costing the Trusts.

One of the major causes of a clinical accident is a breakdown of communication, often through poor record keeping and system failures. We will look at these specifically later in the book.

If a clinical accident occurs then all of the health professionals involved in the care will be accountable and there may be both legal and professional implications. Clinical responsibility cannot be passed like a hot potato. The health professional must take responsibility for all actions that they take and will have to justify the steps taken. It is this foundation that must be grasped at the outset. They cannot avoid responsibility because, for example, they are being supervised, nor can the health professional assume that a consultant in charge of the ward will have to carry that responsibility alone. These complex areas of accountability will be explored in detail later.

In recent years, I have heard that some Trusts advocate a 'no blame' culture. When something has gone wrong the individuals concerned will not carry any blame. Whilst to some extent this may remove the difficulties surrounding the reluctance of staff to come forward to whistle blow and the lack of openness when something has gone wrong, I do not believe that the law would uphold such a culture, as this would remove from the equation the health professional's accountability. My own view is that a more sensible approach would be a 'fair blame' culture. So that those responsible are held to account, but there is not a culture of passing the buck and blaming those who are not responsible. To adopt a 'no-blame' culture may result in inadvertently turning a blind eye to matters of importance and ultimately risk management.

REFERENCE

1 National Health Service Litigation Authority. *Report and Accounts: fact sheet 2, financial information*. London: National Health Service Litigation Authority; 2008.

CHAPTER 2

Accountability

'I was following my orders. My boss told me to do it.'

The concept of 'accountability' is one which is familiar to all health professionals. It is a word that they all know and use and forms part of their working day vocabulary. But how can it be defined?

TASK

1   Before you read further try to define 'accountability'.
2   List the areas where you think you are accountable.

ACCOUNTABILITY IN A LEGAL CONTEXT

In a legal context, there is no distinction between responsibility and accountability. Responsibility can be defined as being accountable for, answerable for or liable to be called to account.

As a health professional, patients must be able to trust you with their lives and health. To justify that trust, care must be the health professional's first concern, providing a good standard of care. Health professionals are personally accountable for their professional practice and must be able to justify their decisions, actions and omissions.

The reality of the situation is that a health professional is, on a personal level, answerable and can be called to account. Once that premise has been accepted, the inevitable and consequent enquiry that must flow from it is to whom and how is that accountability discharged?

It is the courts that determine whether or not a health professional has discharged their duty. The law, by its nature, is reactive and is invoked after the event. It is only when a real case is presented that the judges will deliberate and deliver judgment. It follows then that issues are debated with the benefit of hindsight. Thus, we cannot go to the courts with hypothetical questions or scenarios: 'If I do it in particular way, will I be in trouble?' The usual sequence is that something will have happened to trigger an investigation. This will raise the question of accountability. When the health professional appears before the court his acts or omissions will be weighed up and judgment will be delivered. The practical effect is that health professionals make decisions about patient care and it is hoped that the courts will ultimately support them.

Accountability has now been put into its legal context. The next question then is: to who is the health professional accountable?

TASK

■ To whom are you accountable?

List them

THE FOUR AREAS OF ACCOUNTABILITY

There is not just a single individual or body to whom the health professional is accountable, but four separate and distinct areas where they are answerable. In the widest sense, the health professional is answerable to society. Perhaps, and more importantly from the health professional's perspective, he must be accountable and answerable to the patient. Equally, the health professional will be answerable to their employer and last, but certainly not least, the health professional will also be accountable to his profession.

There is one other area of accountability that might be considered and that is that the health professional is accountable to themselves. This is a moral obligation and one that is not enforced by law, but might be considered as being at the centre of professional practice and skill. However, these moral and ethical considerations are not within the ambit of this book.

Having established that the health professional can be accountable in four quite separate and distinct respects, we need next to examine how that impacts in practice.

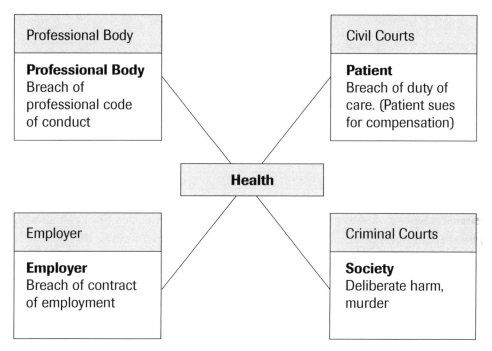

FIGURE 2.1 Four areas of accountability

Society

Health professionals are accountable to society for issues that are in the public interest. Society dictates the kind of behaviour they will or will not tolerate. If someone is murdered, society says this is wrong and the murderer must be punished. Society's view is then enshrined in criminal law. We have seen manslaughter charges brought against school teachers where a child has died on a school trip. These charges are brought because the teachers have not lived up to the trust society bestowed on them. It will be argued that the individual has fallen short of what society accepts and demands of someone in that position. If they are found guilty they face a penalty. As society's values change, the law may change to reflect this. For example, suicide used to be a crime but is no longer, as the law was changed to decriminalise it following the wishes of society.

The kinds of cases that come before the criminal courts involving health professionals include theft, assault and battery, murder, manslaughter or manslaughter through gross negligence. Recently, we have seen consideration given to criminal charges being brought against an NHS chief executive following the investigation into failures at a Trust after poor hygiene standards were linked to patient deaths.

Criminal cases involving health professionals often generate a lot of media attention. They include cases such as Harold Shipman,[1] who was found guilty of the murder of 15 of his patients, Beverly Allitt,[2] who was convicted of the murder and attempted murder of many children, Kevin Cobb,[3] a nurse who was found guilty of drugging three patients and raping two of them and the case of Adomako,[4] where gross professional misconduct constituted the criminal offence of manslaughter.

When dealing with accountability to society the discharge of such accountability rests with the criminal courts. The criminal court acts in the public interest; the prosecutor derives no benefit. Criminal proceedings are brought against an individual. It is personal. It is not possible for the individual to be indemnified by the employer or defence union. The health professional's boss is not able to say 'don't worry I'll serve your prison sentence for you'!

Where, for example, a fine is imposed, the court makes it clear that this to be paid by the individual personally and must not be paid by their employer.

The kinds of sanctions that may be imposed by the criminal courts include:

➤ custodial sentence – imprisonment
➤ fine
➤ community-based sentences.

Any criminal conviction is automatically reported to the professional body of a health professional. It is usual for a health professional to have to report any criminal conviction to their professional body in any event.

Patient

Health professionals are accountable to the patient or client. The discharge of accountability rests with the civil courts; that is the County or High Court. Unlike the criminal process, the civil law is not about punishment. If a patient is injured as a result of negligent treatment the patient may seek financial compensation through the civil courts. The purpose of the patient suing for compensation, referred to by the court as 'damages', is to put them back into the financial position they would have been had the incident not occurred.

EXAMPLE OF COMPENSATION

A patient attends hospital as a day patient for the removal of a mole under general anaesthetic. Due to an error with the records the patient is added to the wrong theatre list and instead of carrying out the removal of the mole, the patient's leg is amputated by mistake. The patient sues for compensation for financial loss.

Had the correct procedure been carried out the patient would have had the mole removed and then been discharged that day. He would have returned to work and usual daily life. However, as a result of the amputation, the patient's condition is such that he has to stay in hospital, cannot return to work (so has lost his income), will require care at home, equipment and further treatment, which he will now have to pay for.

The damages the patient claims are to recompense him for this financial loss. There will also be some recompense for pain and suffering.

The value of such claims will vary as it is based on the loss endured by the individual. Therefore the same identical errors may arise with two patients, but one claim may be valued at £5000 whereas the other might be valued at £5 million. The difference is that if the first patient was unemployed at the time of the incident and never likely to work in any event then there is no claim for loss of earnings. Whereas the second patient may be a professional footballer at the peak of his career and therefore the loss of earnings could be very substantial.

A patient cannot sue for compensation simply because there has been an adverse outcome. There are many issues that have to be established for a claim by the patient to succeed. The onus is upon them to establish the legal principles. They have to establish all of the following:

1 that the defendant owed the claimant a duty of care
2 that the defendant breached that duty of care
3 that such breach 'caused' the injury or loss (known as causation)
4 that the injury was 'reasonably foreseeable'
5 and that as a result the claimant has suffered loss.

The civil process, duty of care and how to quantify a claim are discussed in more detail in a later chapter.

If a patient sues for compensation they will usually sue the Trust. This has the effect that the health professional that caused the harm does not have to pay the compensation themselves. This is because of the relationship with the employer of 'vicarious liability', which is discussed below. Although the health professional does not pay the compensation themselves, this does not mean they are exonerated from responsibility. Indeed, the health professional will be accountable to his employer and the other areas of accountability.

If a patient brings a claim in the civil court the health professionals involved in their care would have to give evidence. They would have to give an account of what happened and would have to prepare a witness statement for this purpose.

Employer

Vicarious liability

If a patient has been injured as a result of negligence then the patient may sue for compensation. Who does the patient sue? Does he sue the individual health professional, the Trust or both?

Some employers accept liability for the negligent acts and/or omissions of their employees. This is known as 'vicarious liability'. Such cover does not normally extend to activities undertaken outside the health professional's employment. Independent practice would not normally be covered by vicarious liability.

If a health professional is self-employed or works in the private health sector it is the individual health professional's responsibility to establish their insurance status. In situations where employers do not accept vicarious liability, it is recommended that health professionals should obtain adequate professional indemnity insurance. If a health professional is unable to secure professional indemnity insurance, they will need to demonstrate that all their clients/patients are fully informed of this fact and the implications this might have in the event of a claim by the client/patient for negligence.

Where the employer is vicariously liable for the employee they are liable for the employee's acts and omissions. It does not matter whether the employee is full-time, part-time, temporary or agency staff – they will be considered as acting as an agent for the Trust. In practical terms, this means the Trust is responsible for the actions of their employees. It therefore follows that although the individual health professional may have been negligent, any claim for compensation will be met by the employer. Whilst there is nothing in law preventing the patient from suing the individual health professionals, the patient will usually choose to sue the Trust rather than the individuals. This is because it is an easier process and the Trust is more likely to have the financial resources to pay out the compensation. There is no point in suing a man of straw (someone with no money).

When a patient sues for compensation it is usually the Trust and not the individual that is sued, so if the patient's claim is successful, the Trust pays the compensation. Thus, the health professionals concerned in the incident do not themselves have to pay the compensation. However, there are exceptions to this. The Trust may, in certain circumstances, seek to recoup from the individuals concerned in the incident any compensation the Trust has paid out. This, however, should only be pursued in exceptional circumstances. Exceptional circumstances are likely to include causing deliberate harm, such as the Beverly Allitt[5] case. However, the Nursing and Midwifery Council (NMC)[6] warns that where a nurse prescribes outside their powers the Trust may not stand by them. Therefore it is recommended that health professionals have indemnity insurance in the event that a claim is made personally against the health professional.

The Trust sought to recover from Beverly Allitt[7] the compensation paid out to the victims. In reality of course the Trust is unlikely to recover the compensation from her. As she is in prison she has no income and is therefore unlikely to have the means to pay back the money. One of the reasons why a Trust may seek to recover compensation from the individual is to satisfy public perception. They do not want the public to think that they are condoning this kind of behaviour. Justice must be seen to be done.

Breach of contract

Notwithstanding that it is the Trust, not the individual, that will be sued and that it is the Trust that will pay out the compensation, this does not fully exonerate the health professionals and they are still accountable to their employer.

The employer may be displeased about what has happened and it is open to the employer to look into the matter. The employer will examine the case alongside the contract of employment to see whether there has been any breach of that contract, and whether the employee acted outside their job description.

EXAMPLE OF BREACH OF CONTRACT

A district nurse had worked for many years in community care. She took up a new post with a Trust in the A&E department of a hospital. The standard job description was that only a doctor can suture hands and face. A patient was admitted whose face required suturing. The nurse considered herself far more experienced than the junior doctors, so she did suture the patient's face. It went wrong and the patient was left with scarring that could have been avoided. The employer considered that the nurse was in breach of her contract of employment. The job description was clear: she was prohibited from suturing a patient's face. The employer dismissed the nurse from employment.

It is implied in a contract of employment that an employee will obey the reasonable instructions of the employer and that the employee will use all their care and skill in carrying out their duties. As an employee the health professional must have regard to their roles and responsibilities and cannot embark on a frolic of their own. They are answerable to the employer and it is open to the employer to look at a situation and address it.

The kinds of sanctions the employer can invoke are:

➤ grievance procedure
➤ disciplinary procedure.

This could lead to:

➤ warning
➤ demotion
➤ suspension
➤ dismissal.

Health professionals are answerable to their employer and this may result in disciplinary action with sanctions. The ultimate sanction is, of course, dismissal.

Professional body

Professional bodies regulate health professionals. Their primary aim is to protect the public. This is achieved by setting and maintaining standards of education, training, conduct and performance, which the public is entitled to expect. These are usually set out in the codes of conduct.

It is the responsibility of the health professionals to be familiar with their codes of conduct and the duties of a health professional.

Professional bodies will look at whether the health professional has maintained their professional duty and will expect their members to uphold its professional standards. They will look at whether the health professional is competent to practice, whether they are safe to practice, whether they have maintained professional standards and so on.

Information about a health professional may be received by the professional body from a number of sources. Anyone has the right to make a complaint. It there is a criminal conviction this will be reported to the professional body. Non-criminal misconduct may also be reported. A health professional may be referred to his professional body by a judge following a civil court hearing. The police may report the conduct of a health professional. A patient or their family, the employer, managers, colleagues or other health professionals may report them. The professional body will then investigate the matter and this may result in a hearing before a conduct and competence committee to make a decision.

There are many regulatory bodies governing healthcare, including:
- Nursing and Midwifery Council (NMC)[8]
- General Medical Council (GMC)[9]
- General Dental Council (GDC)[10]
- General Chiropractic Council (GCC)[11]
- General Optical Council (GOC)[12]
- Health Professions Council (HPC).[13]

Professional bodies will be concerned with issues surrounding fitness to practice and the health professional's suitability to be on the register without restrictions. They will consider whether the health professional's fitness to practice is impaired. Many matters that are heard before the conduct and competency committees include performing below the standards required, failure to maintain adequate records, failure to maintain adequate and accurate reports and failure to maintain effective communication to service users, relatives and other professionals.

Issues that can impair fitness to practice will include:

a **Lack of competence.**

For example:
— persistent lack of ability in correctly and/or appropriately calculating, administering and recording the administration or disposal of medicines

— persistent lack of ability in properly identifying care needs and, accordingly

— planning and delivering appropriate care.

b **Physical or mental ill health.**

For example:

— alcohol or drug dependence

— untreated serious mental illness.

c **Misconduct.**

For example:

— physical or verbal abuse

— theft

— deliberate failure to deliver adequate care

— deliberate failure to keep proper records.

d **A finding by any other health or social care regulator or licensing body that the registered professional's fitness to practise is impaired.**

e **A conviction or caution (including a finding of guilt by a court martial).**

For example:

— theft

— fraud or other dishonest activities

— violence

— sexual offences

— accessing or downloading child pornography or other illegal material from the internet

— illegally dealing or importing drugs.

f **Fraudulent or incorrect entry in the professional register.**

Sanctions

There are sanctions that can be imposed by the professional bodies. The purpose of such sanctions is not to punish the health professional, but to protect the public.

The kind of sanctions that can be imposed include:

➤ a conditions of practice order; for example, they may impose conditions that the health professional must comply with, for example they may require them to undertake training or work with supervision

➤ a caution order

➤ a suspension order

➤ a striking-off order.

Outside professional duties

Health professionals also need to be aware that regulatory bodies can look outside what they do in their professional roles as to whether they are fit to practice.

> **The NMC guidelines state that:**
> 'You must uphold the reputation of your profession at all times.'

Examples of health professionals who have been removed from the register or had other sanctions imposed for matters outside their role as a health professional include:

➤ a nurse soliciting for the purpose of prostitution
➤ a paramedic removed from the register of the HPC for having been convicted of driving a motor vehicle under the influence of alcohol.

Although the offence was committed when the health professional was off duty, members of the public place their trust in health professionals and are entitled to expect that health professionals will conduct themselves in a professional manner.

Offences like these, however isolated they may be, undermine public confidence in the health professionals. The health professional's behaviour demonstrates that their conduct falls short of the standards of personal conduct expected of a registered health professional.

The healthcare professional can be called to account in all four areas of accountability, which means, in effect, they can be tried four times.

The case of Beverly Allitt is an illustration of this.[14]

Society – Beverly Allitt was accountable to society. She was considered to have failed society, committing criminal offences in killing and injuring children. For this she was prosecuted in the criminal courts and a custodial sentence was imposed.

Patient – Beverly Allitt was accountable to the patients. The parents of the deceased and injured children brought civil claims for compensation and the Trust paid out compensation.

Employer – Her employers pursued disciplinary proceedings against her and she was dismissed from her employment.

Professional body – The professional body removed her from the register.

Where a health professional is not a member of a professional body, such as a healthcare assistant, they should still follow professional standards and they will still be answerable in the other areas of accountability.

It is important for health professionals to appreciate that the four areas of accountability are separate and distinct. Where, for example, due to lack of resources, the Trust condones or turns a blind eye to the carrying out of duties that are beyond the skill of the health professional, the Trust may decide to take no disciplinary action. However, the Trust cannot protect the health professional from the other areas of accountability. So, if the patient was harmed despite the Trust having turned a blind eye the patient can still sue, criminal charges can be brought against the health professionals and the professional body can step in. It is no defence for the health professional to say 'the Trust knew about it'. The health professional will still be held accountable for their actions.

It does not necessarily follow that if an employer dismisses the health professional, the professional body will strike a health professional from the register. Nor does it necessarily follow that if the professional body strikes someone from the register, they will be dismissed from their employment. However, in these circumstances, the health professional concerned would lose their registered position.

Recap
The four areas of accountability are:
1 society
2 patient
3 employer
4 professional body.

REFERENCES
1 R v Harold Shipman 2000. www.the-shipman-inquiry.org.uk/trialday.asp?Day=58 (accessed 3 April 2009).
2 R v Beverly Allitt 1992 [2007] EWHC 2845 (QB).
3 *Male nurse used sedative to kill and rape*; www.guardian.co.uk/Archive/Article/0,4273, 4019340,00.html (accessed 3 April 2009).
4 R v Adomako 1995 1 AC 171; 1994 3 All ER 79.
5 R v Beverly Allitt, op. cit. www.judiciary.gov.uk/docs/judgments_guidance/allitt_061207. pdf (accessed 3 April 2009).
6 www.nmc-uk.org
7 R v Beverly Allitt, op. cit.

8 www.nmc-uk.org
9 www.gmc-uk.org
10 www.gdc-uk.org
11 www.gcc-uk.org
12 www.optical.org
13 www.hpc-uk.org
14 R v Beverly Allitt, op. cit.

CHAPTER 3

Clinical responsibility and the law

We have already looked at the four areas of accountability: society, the patient, the employer and the professional body.

In order to put clinical responsibility into context, it is important for the health professional to understand the many different factors that have an effect on them. These include how accountability is discharged, the court process, the components of a legal claim for compensation, the duty of care, how this duty is measured and also how issues like waiting lists, lack of resources and following orders will affect them. This will help to put clinical responsibility in context.

We will now look at the court process.

THE LEGAL SYSTEM

Health professionals may become involved in the court process when an issue of their accountability arises. The discharge of accountability rests ultimately with the court. A health professional may have to give evidence in court, for example, when there has been a serious untoward incident. The kind of court proceedings in which a health professional may become involved can include an inquest, civil proceedings for compensation, criminal proceedings for gross negligence, professional conduct hearing or employment tribunal for breach of contract.

LEGAL PERSONNEL

In England and Wales, there is a division of legal personnel into solicitors and barristers. There is a popular misconception that a lawyer begins his professional career as a solicitor and, if he is good enough, he then moves on to become a barrister. This is not so. These are different professions and a choice of which profession to pursue must be made at the start of his legal career. The training is different for each profession.

The solicitor, following completion of their law degree (or equivalent), must then go on to complete the Law Society finals (legal practice course [LPC]) and undertake two years in practice under a training contract. They are then admitted onto the Roll of Solicitors.

To become a barrister, following their law degree, the aspiring lawyer sits the bar final examinations and then undertakes six months in practice under the guidance of another barrister. They are a pupil to that barrister and the position is called a pupilage.

After a period in practice, both solicitors and barristers can re-train to change professions. The word 'lawyer' is the generic term for those who practice law.

Solicitor

Solicitors are members of the Law Society and have a practising certificate that is renewed every year.

A solicitor has the hands-on day-to-day contact with the client. They carry out the investigations, collect all of the evidence, prepare the documentation and get the case ready for trial.

Solicitors have rights of audience in the lower courts, such as the Magistrates Court and County Court. 'Rights of audience' means that they undertake advocacy; that is, they present the case on behalf of one party. This means that where a case goes to trial in the Magistrates or County Court the solicitor will deal with the entire case, from first contact with the client through to its conclusion at court.

Solicitors do not automatically have rights of audience in the High Court and Crown Court but they can take certification to give them this right of audience. Where the solicitor does not have rights of audience in court then a barrister is instructed to undertake the advocacy in court.

Barrister (counsel)

Barristers are also referred to as 'counsel'. They are members of The General Council of the Bar (Bar Council).

Barristers undertake the advocacy, but they do not become involved in the day-to-day litigation. Usually the solicitor will prepare the case and once it is ready for trial they will instruct the barrister to present the case before the judge at the trial.

The barrister may, however, be instructed by the solicitor during the course of a case in order to advise them on certain legal issues. They will sometimes hold a conference with the solicitor and the experts to look at the legal issues before a case goes to trial. The advice may be oral at the conference and/or in writing. The barrister may also assist in drafting certain court documentation, such as the statement of a claim or a defence.

Barristers are independent sole practitioners who are usually self-employed and work out of 'chambers', which is another name for their office. Although they can be employed by law firms or other organisations, they cannot form partnerships.

Legal executives

Legal executives are qualified lawyers specialising in a particular area of law.

They will have passed the Institute of Legal Executives (ILEX)[1] Professional Qualification in Law in an area of legal practice to the same level as that required of solicitors. They will have at least five years experience of working under the supervision of a solicitor in legal practice or the legal department of a private company or local/national government.

They are issued with an annual practising certificate, and only Fellows of ILEX may describe themselves as 'legal executives'. Their day-to-day work is similar to that of a solicitor. They handle various legal aspects and are involved in actions in the courts.

Legal executives are fee earners – in private practice their work is charged directly to clients – making a direct contribution to the income of a law firm. This is an important difference between legal executives and other types of legal support staff who tend to handle work of a more routine nature. However, they cannot become partners in firms.

Coroner

The coroner is an independent judicial officer presiding over the Coroner's Court.

The coroner has a duty to investigate the circumstances of sudden, unnatural or uncertified deaths that are reported to him. He has to find out the medical cause of the death, if it is not known, and to enquire about the cause of it – if it was due to violence or was otherwise unnatural. In addition, the coroner is responsible for determining issues of treasure trove.

Deaths will usually be reported to the coroner by the police, a doctor or a registrar of births and deaths. This can happen when no doctor has treated the deceased during his or her last illness or when the death was sudden, unexpected or unnatural. Even where a death has been reported, the coroner may decide, after preliminary questioning, that death was quite natural and the investigation should go no further.

Where a death has been reported to the coroner the deceased will be moved to the mortuary at a local hospital. The deceased is then under the coroner's jurisdiction and will remain so until the coroner releases the body for the funeral arrangements to be made.

Post-mortems

If the coroner decides that a medical examination of the deceased is required, a pathologist will carry out a post mortem. If the post mortem shows the death to have been a natural one, there may be no need for an inquest; however, if the death is not due to a natural cause then the coroner will hold an inquest.

Inquests

An inquest is not a trial, it is an inquiry to find out who has died, and how, when and where they died. It is not the job of the coroner to blame anyone for the death, as a trial would do.

Most inquests are held without a jury. There are particular reasons when a jury will be called, including if the death occurred in prison, in police custody or if the death resulted from an incident at work. In this case, it is the jury and not the coroner, which makes the final decision (this is called returning the verdict). Jurors are paid expenses and some money towards loss of earnings.

It is not the role of the coroner to apportion blame as to who caused the death. This would be established at a trial through the criminal or civil courts.

Lawyers

The term 'lawyer' is used loosely to refer to a broad variety of legally trained personnel. It includes barristers, solicitors, legal executives and people who are involved with the law but do not practice it on behalf of individual clients, such as judges, law clerks and legislators.

SOURCES OF LAW

We know the law exists, but we do not often think about it in our everyday lives even though it is continuously in operation, for example, when goods are bought and sold, when people get married or companies are formed. The law lays down rules in respect of all of these matters. When things are done in the usual way there is little reason to worry. In the normal course of events people only begin to consider the law when some uncertainty or difficulty arises. When a person looks into their situation after a difficulty has arisen they may find it is probably too late. The law, by its nature, applies retrospectively. It is usually when something has gone wrong that the law steps in.

Everyday decisions are made about patient care, planning and treatment. Health professionals go about their daily routines and whilst terms like 'accountability' and 'responsibility' form part of their everyday vocabulary they do not sit back and think 'what does it really mean'? But when something goes wrong they become accountable. By its nature accountability applies retrospectively. The discharge of accountability rests with the courts. The health professional cannot go the courts beforehand and say 'if I do something in this way, will I be in trouble'? In reality they go about the daily tasks weighing up risks and making decisions and hope that when they do so, the courts, the employer and the professional body will uphold what they do. Being forewarned is being forearmed and understanding the law and accountability will help the health professional make the right decisions.

The health professional must know the area of law that affects them. For example, those working in mental health should be familiar with the Mental Health Act 1983,[2] Mental Capacity Act 2005[3] and other legislation. Remember, ignorance of the law is no defence.

Very broadly speaking, the law is a set of rules. The law in England and Wales is made up of statutes and common law. ('Common law' is sometimes referred to as 'case law'.)

STATUTES

A statute is law set out in an Act of Parliament, declaring, commanding or prohibiting something. It identifies the purpose of the law, how it is to be interpreted, penalties for failure to adhere to the law and the remedies available to an injured party.

The courts apply a statute to the circumstances in determining whether there has been a breach of the law and then apply the penalties.

Here is an extract from a statute, the Mental Capacity Act 2005.[4]

MENTAL CAPACITY ACT 2005
PART 1

PERSONS WHO LACK CAPACITY
The principles

1 The principles

(1) The following principles apply for the purposes of this Act.

(2) A person must be assumed to have capacity unless it is established that he lacks capacity.

(3) A person is not to be treated as unable to make a decision unless all practicable steps to help him to do so have been taken without success.

(4) A person is not to be treated as unable to make a decision merely because he makes an unwise decision.

(5) An act done, or decision made, under this Act for or on behalf of a person who lacks capacity must be done, or made, in his best interests.

(6) Before the act is done, or the decision is made, regard must be had to whether the purpose for which it is needed can be as effectively achieved in a way that is less restrictive of the person's rights and freedom of action.

44 Ill-treatment or Neglect

(1) Subsection (2) applies if a person ('D') –

   (a) has the care of a person ('P') who lacks, or whom D reasonably believes to lack, capacity

   (b) is the donee of a lasting power of attorney, or an enduring power of attorney (within the meaning of Schedule 4), created by P, or

   (c) is a deputy appointed by the court for P.

(2) D is guilty of an offence if he ill-treats or wilfully neglects P.

---

(3)   A person guilty of an offence under this section is liable –
  (a)   on summary conviction, to imprisonment for a term not exceeding 12 months or a fine not exceeding the statutory maximum or both;
  (b)   on conviction on indictment, to imprisonment for a term not exceeding 5 years or a fine or both.

A statute sets out the law. For example, take a look at the extracts from the Mental Capacity Act 2005. Section 1 of the Act sets out the principles that a person is presumed to have capacity unless it is established that the person lacks capacity. It also states that a person should not be treated as unable to make a decision merely because he makes an unwise decision.

Section 44 of the Act has the effect that a person is guilty of an offence if he ill-treats or wilfully neglects the person and that the offence is punishable by a fine or imprisonment for a term not exceeding five years or both.

Statute and clinical responsibility

In relation to clinical responsibility, although there is no statute specifically dealing with purely clinical responsibility there are, however, statutes that impact on and apply to it.

Examples of statutes that impact on clinical responsibility include:
➤ Human Rights Act 1998[5]
➤ Mental Health Act 1983[6]
➤ Freedom of Information Act 2000[7]
➤ Data Protection Act 1998[8]
➤ Access to Health Records Act 1990.[9]

COMMON LAW (CASE LAW)

Where no statute exists, the courts develop law by considering the particular set of circumstances in a case and making a decision. Those decisions become the law – hence the term 'case law'. Another term for this is 'common law'. Important decisions, together with reasons for their decisions, are recorded in law reports. These decisions are then followed by the courts when dealing with cases in similar circumstances. They are followed as legal precedents.

If the common law differs from a statute, the statute will overrule the common law.

An example of what a law report looks like is set out in the extract below: Chester v Afshar House of Lords 2004.[10]

JUDGMENTS – CHESTER (RESPONDENT) V. AFSHAR (APPELLANT)

HOUSE OF LORDS SESSION 2003–04 [2004] UKHL 41
on appeal from: [2002] EWCA Civ 724

HOUSE OF LORDS
OPINIONS OF THE LORDS OF APPEAL FOR JUDGMENT
IN THE CAUSE
Chester (Respondent) v. Afshar (Appellant)
[2004] UKHL 41
LORD BINGHAM OF CORNHILL

My Lords

1 The central question in this appeal is whether the conventional approach to causation in negligence actions should be varied where the claim is based on a doctor's negligent failure to warn a patient of a small but unavoidable risk of surgery when, following surgery performed with due care and skill, such risk eventuates but it is not shown that, if duly warned, the patient would not have undergone surgery with the same small but unavoidable risk of mishap. Is it relevant to the outcome of the claim to decide whether, duly warned, the patient probably would or probably would not have consented to undergo the surgery in question?

2 I am indebted to my noble and learned friend Lord Hope of Craighead for his detailed account of the facts and the history of these proceedings, which I need not repeat.

3 For some six years beginning in 1988 the claimant, Miss Chester, suffered repeated episodes of low back pain. She was conservatively treated by Dr Wright, a consultant rheumatologist, who administered epidural and sclerosant injections. An MRI scan in 1992 showed evidence of disc protrusions. In 1994, on the eve of a professional trip abroad, Miss Chester suffered another episode of pain and disability: she could 'hardly walk', and had reduced control of her bladder. Dr Wright gave another epidural injection, and Miss Chester was able to make the trip, using a wheelchair at Heathrow.

But after the trip the pain returned. A further MRI scan revealed marked protrusion of discs into the spinal canal. After further conservative treatment which proved ineffective, Dr Wright referred Miss Chester to Mr Afshar, a distinguished consultant neurosurgeon with much experience of disc surgery, although Miss Chester was understandably reluctant to undergo surgery if this could be avoided.

REFERENCES

1 www.ilex.org.uk
2 Mental Health Act 1983.
3 Mental Capacity Act 2005.
4 Ibid.
5 Human Rights Act 1998.
6 Mental Health Act, op. cit.
7 Freedom of Information Act 2000.
8 Data Protection Act 1998.
9 Access to Health Records Act 1990.
10 Chester v Afshar House of Lords [2004] HL 41; [2005] 1 AC 134; [2004] 3 WLR 927; [2004] 4 All ER 587.

CHAPTER 4

Court system

The law is made up of statute law and case law. Breach of either may give rise to civil or criminal liability.

Here is a simplified illustration of the court structure (*see* Figure 4.1). Within the court structure there are a variety of branches not illustrated here, such as family division, tribunals and public inquiries.

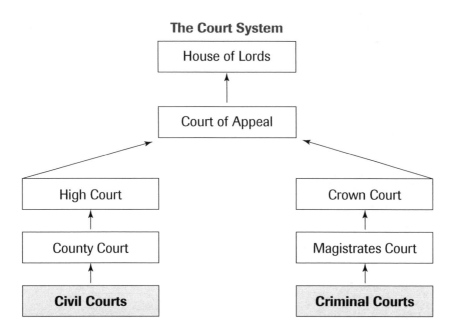

FIGURE 4.1 The court system

THE ADVERSARIAL AND INQUISITORIAL PROCESS

The court system in England and Wales, Scotland and Northern Ireland is adversarial – a system that has been imported in many countries all over the world. What this means in practice is that during the court hearing at trial there will be at least two parties each with a different version of events and the system places the parties in opposition to each other in order to decide who has the best evidence and which party can prove its case. The judge, the jury and/or the adjudicator hear all sides and then reach a decision. This is the same for almost all court forums and so includes criminal, civil, professional conduct and tribunal hearings.

The only time this differs is at an inquest in the Coroner's Court, which is inquisitorial. The reason why this differs from the adversarial process is that it is an inquiry – the purpose of which is to determine the cause of death and not to apportion blame. However, the lawyers do adopt an adversarial approach at inquests as well.

CORONER'S COURT

Death of a patient

A health professional during the course of their work may encounter the death of the patient. This can be distressing and this distress may be compounded by numerous questions from troubled relatives. From the relatives' point of view this may be the first time they have had to deal with a death and they will be looking to the health professional for advice and guidance. It is important that the health professional has knowledge of procedures and the law so that they can answer any questions.

Following the Shipman Inquiry, recommendations were made in respect of certification of death and the procedures for inquest in Coroner's Courts.[1]

The law requires that certification of the death must be undertaken by a doctor (of medicine). A nurse may, however, verify a death – provided they are appropriately trained. The Nursing and Midwifery Council (NMC) has provided advice on verification of death by registered nurses.[2] A registered nurse may confirm or verify death has occurred, providing the local protocol allows such an action. The protocol should include guidance on when other authorities, e.g. the police or the coroner, should be informed prior to removal of the body. Where a nurse verifies the death, education is necessary to ensure they have the confidence, competence, knowledge and skills to equip them for undertaking this role. Their record should document the actions they have taken, the date and time of death and any other information required by the hospital policy.

The general office of the hospital or the medical records department discusses with the bereaved relatives the administrative details that must be dealt with. However, at night, at weekends or bank holidays, the nurse may have to deal with the administrative details and should therefore be familiar with the issues relating to the registration of death and disposal of the body.

Deaths that have to be reported to the coroner
Circumstances in which deaths have to be reported to the coroner are:
1 where there is reasonable cause to suspect a person has died a violent or unnatural death
2 when there is reasonable cause to suspect a person has died of an unknown cause
3 the person has died in prison or in such place or under such circumstances as to require an inquest.

The causes of death to be reported to the coroner include: maternal deaths during abortions, accidents and injuries, alcoholism, anaesthetics and operations, crime or suspected crime, drugs, ill-treatment, industrial diseases, infant deaths if in any way obscure, pensioners where death might be connected with pensionable disability, persons in legal custody, poisoning, septicaemia if originating from injury, and stillbirth where there is the possibility or suspicion that the child may have been born alive.

If it is likely to be a case that goes before the coroner then no beneficial post-mortem should be undertaken without the coroner's approval. The coroner can order a post-mortem examination to be carried out before deciding to hold an inquest.

Post-mortems
The coroner may instruct that a post-mortem be carried out to determine the cause of death. Where the coroner makes an order for post-mortem then the person in possession of the body has no choice but to agree.

Medical staff may sometimes request that the relatives' permission be obtained. However, the relatives have no right to refuse. (Consent of the relatives should be obtained where there is retention of organs for the purpose of research.)[3]

The inquest

At an inquest the coroner presides over the whole proceedings. The coroner decides which evidence to hear and which witnesses to call. The coroner then hears the evidence and makes a decision. The reason why this differs from the adversarial process is that it is an inquiry – the purpose of which is to determine the cause of death and not to apportion blame. However, those who have given evidence in the Coroner's Court will know that the system feels the same because there is usually representation for the deceased and representation for the Trust. In fact, it can feel worse because in the other courts the lawyers know the rules; they know the kind of questions that they can ask. In the Coroner's Court, the coroner will sometimes invite the family to ask questions. The family are not aware of the rules and boundaries and will sometimes come out with a blunt question such as 'why did you kill my mother?'

The purpose of the inquest is to determine the cause of death and the coroner will be annoyed if the lawyers use this process as a fishing expedition to obtain information to establish blame.

An application to the High Court can be made to challenge a decision by the coroner not to hold an inquest.

CASE

R (on the application of Touche) v. HM Coroner for Inner North London (2001)[4]

A mother had suffered from a cerebral haemorrhage soon after giving birth in circumstances that suggested that had her blood pressure been properly monitored immediately after birth, her death might have been avoided. The coroner concluded that she had suffered a natural death. The High Court adjudicated that the coroner had made an error in deciding not to hold an inquest. The coroner appealed to the Court of Appeal, who dismissed the appeal. The Court of Appeal held that for the purpose of the Coroners Act 1988 section 1(1) (a),[5] a death by natural causes was an 'unnatural death', which was wholly unexpected and would not have occurred but for some culpable human failing.

Purpose of the inquest

The purpose of an inquest is not to apportion blame but to ascertain:

1 the identity of the deceased

2 how, where and when the deceased came by his death
3 the particulars, to be registered concerning the death.

The Coroners Act 1988 section 11(6)[6] specifically states that the purpose of the proceedings shall not include a finding of any person guilty of murder, manslaughter or infanticide.

Who should attend an inquest?
Pursuant to The Coroners Act 1988 section 11(2),[7] the coroner has a duty to examine under oath anyone who has knowledge of the facts whom he considers it to be appropriate to examine. The coroner has considerable discretion in deciding who should attend. The coroner must notify the date, time and place of the inquest to the spouse or near relatives or personal representative of the deceased and any other person who may have caused or contributed to the death of the deceased, or a person appointed by a trade union where death may have been caused by industrial disease or an injury received at work.

A health professional who has been involved in the care of a patient who has died may be required to give evidence at an inquest. They will be asked to give an account of what happened by way of a witness statement and they will be required to attend the inquest to give oral evidence.

CRIMINAL COURTS
Criminal courts deal with criminal matters. Situations giving rise to criminal charges in relation to healthcare may include causing deliberate harm to a patient; for example, the cases of Beverly Allitt[8] who was convicted of murder and attempted murder of many children, Harold Shipman[9] who was found guilty of the murder of 15 of his patients and Kevin Cobb,[10] a nurse who was found guilty of drugging three patients and raping two of them. Other matters that come before the criminal courts include manslaughter for gross negligence or recklessness, arising out of gross professional misconduct (R v Adomako),[11] assault and battery, fraud or theft (R v Beverly Allit 1992).[12]

Prior to a matter coming before the court an investigation is carried out.

Investigation and decision to prosecute
The police will decide whether criminal charges will be brought. They will carry out an investigation and as part of that investigation the health

professional will be interviewed by the police to give a full explanation of what happened. The police, when carrying out their investigations by questioning during interviews, including searching premises for evidence and securing and gathering evidence, have to comply with the rules and guidelines under the Police and Criminal Evidence Act 1984, PACE.[13]

The health professional may be asked to accompany the police to the police station and they may be interviewed there. They may be arrested before they are taken to the police station or they may be arrested later whilst at the police station. If the health professional is arrested then a caution must be given and the health professional is entitled to have legal representation. The caution should be given as soon as they are arrested for an offence and before being questioned about the offence for the purpose of obtaining evidence that may be given to a court in any prosecution.

The next stage is that the health professional may be charged with an offence, cautioned or allowed to leave without charge.

The Crown Prosecution Service (CPS)

The Crown Prosecution Service (CPS) is responsible for prosecuting criminal cases investigated by the police in England and Wales. In Scotland, the equivalent is the Prosecutor Fiscal's Office. They will consider whether there is sufficient evidence to bring a prosecution.

If it is determined that there is sufficient evidence then the matter will proceed to a trial. The criterion is usually that the CPS believes that there is at least a 50% likelihood of securing a conviction.

The witness

In order to prevent unnecessary anxiety to the health professional they must be aware that they may be interviewed by the police as a witness rather than as an accused person. In these circumstances they are merely assisting the police in their investigation by providing facts. They are not being arrested or charged with an offence and they do not need legal representation. This process may, nevertheless, feel intimidating and they may get some support from the Trust or employer in these circumstances, such as a manager attending the interview with them.

Types of criminal courts

The criminal courts are divided into two strands, the Magistrates Court and the Crown Court. All criminal cases begin in the Magistrates Court (*see* Figure 4.2).

In criminal proceedings, the person being tried is known as the 'defendant' and the people bringing the action against them are called the 'prosecution'. The prosecuting party is usually the CPS, although private prosecutions can also be brought by individuals in certain circumstances.

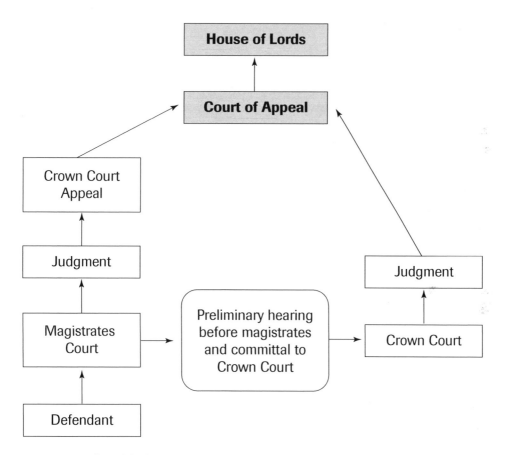

FIGURE 4.2 Simplified version of the criminal court structure

Magistrates Court

All criminal cases begin in the Magistrates Court. The less serious offences are handled entirely in the Magistrates Court. Over 95% of all cases are dealt with in this way. The more serious offences are passed on to the Crown Court.

Cases in the Magistrates Court are heard either by three lay magistrates or one District Judge. The lay magistrates, or 'Justices of the Peace', as they are also known, are local people who volunteer their services. They are unpaid except for their expenses, do not have formal legal qualifications and are given legal and procedural advice by qualified clerks. District Judges are legally qualified, paid, full-time professional lawyers and are usually based in the larger cities.

Magistrates deal with three kinds of cases.

1 **Summary offences.** These are less serious cases, such as motoring offences and minor assaults, where the defendant is not entitled to trial by jury.

2 **Either-way offences.** As the name implies, these can be dealt with either by the magistrates or before a judge and jury at the Crown Court. Such offences include theft and handling stolen goods. A suspect can insist on their right to trial in the Crown Court. Similarly, magistrates can decide that a case is sufficiently serious that it should be dealt with in the Crown Court – which can impose tougher punishments. A defendant may wish to choose one court over the other because, for example, they may feel that they would get a fairer trial if the matter were to be heard by a jury in the Crown Court rather than by three magistrates in the Magistrates Court.

3 **Indictable-only offences.** For example, murder, manslaughter, rape and robbery; these must be heard at a Crown Court.

For 'summary' offences and for 'either way' offences heard in the magistrates court under 1 and 2 above, if the defendant pleads guilty or if they are later found to be guilty, the magistrates can impose a sentence of up to six months imprisonment or a fine of up to £5000.

If the defendant is found not guilty (also known as 'acquitted'), they are judged innocent in the eyes of the law and should be free to go – provided there are no other cases outstanding against them.

If the case is an indictable-only offence, under 3 above, the involvement of the Magistrates Court is brief. The case will be passed to the Crown Court. This is called a 'committal hearing'. This means that provided there is sufficient evidence against the defendant the case is committed to the Crown Court. At the Magistrates Court a decision will be made on whether to grant bail and on other legal issues in the meantime before the matter is heard in the Crown Court.

In certain circumstances, the defendant may appeal against their conviction or sentence imposed by the magistrates. They will appeal to a single judge sitting in the Crown Court. If they are not satisfied with the Crown Court decision, in certain circumstances they may be able to appeal further to the Court of Appeal and then further to the House of Lords.

Crown Court

Due to the seriousness of offences tried in the Crown Court, these trials take place with a judge and jury.

The Crown Court deals with:

1 indictable-only offences such as murder, manslaughter, rape and robbery
2 either-way offences transferred from the Magistrates Court
3 appeals from the Magistrates Court
4 sentencing decisions transferred from the Magistrates Court. This can happen if the magistrates decide, once they have heard the details of a case, that it warrants a tougher sentence than they are allowed to impose.

If the defendant is found not guilty, they are discharged and no conviction is recorded against their name.

In certain circumstances, as mentioned earlier, once again the defendant may appeal against their conviction or sentence. They will appeal to the Court of Appeal. If they are not satisfied with the Court of Appeal decision they may be able to appeal further to the House of Lords.

The Old Bailey

You may wonder why some high profile cases are heard in the Central Criminal Court otherwise known as the 'The Old Bailey'. The Old Bailey is actually a Crown Court by another name.

Historically, 'The Old Bailey' was considered to be very compact and secure. You could be detained there between the time of the committal and trial; you could be tried there, sentenced there, condemned to the cells there and comfortably hanged and buried there without having to leave the building, except for the purpose of going on to the scaffold!

Nowadays, because of the high level of security facilities it accommodates, this court is used for the most serious and high profile cases.

Sanctions imposed by the courts

When deciding what sentence to impose, magistrates and judges have to take account of both the facts of the case and the circumstances of the offender.

A sentence needs to:

1 protect the public
2 punish the offender fairly and appropriately
3 encourage the offender to make amends for their crime
4 contribute to crime reduction by reducing the chances of the defendant reoffending.

The courts can impose four levels of sentence, depending on the seriousness of the offence:

1 discharges
2 fines
3 community sentences
4 imprisonment.

Fines are the most common option used by the courts. Community sentences can include 'restorative justice' – making amends directly to the victims of crime. The most severe punishment – imprisonment – is generally only used for the most serious offences.

If a crime is an imprisonable offence, it will have a maximum term laid down by Parliament. Judges and magistrates are also given sentencing guidelines, which are designed to provide consistency throughout the criminal justice process. There are also fixed minimum sentences for some serious repeat offenders.

The jury

At the Crown Court the hearing is presided over by a judge and jury in England and Wales. The jury consists of 12 people taken from all walks of life.

When all the evidence has been given to the court the judge will explain the law and summarise the facts of the case to the jury. The jury will then reach a verdict on the innocence or guilt of the defendant. The decision must be unanimous, which means all 12 jurors must agree on the guilt of the defendant for them to be found guilty. If the jury cannot agree then the judge may direct that there can be a majority verdict of 10–12 in order for the defendant to be found guilty. This means that at least 10 people out of the 12 jury members must find the defendant guilty in order for the defendant to be found guilty. This is because of the burden of proof. The prosecution must show beyond a reasonable doubt that the defendant is guilty of a crime. It is a high threshold.

Burden of proof

In criminal cases the burden of proof is 'beyond reasonable doubt'. The jury must be sure of the guilt of the defendant. The standard of proof is higher in criminal cases than civil cases because somebody's liberty is at stake, so the court has to be sure that an offence had been committed. It is up to the prosecution to prove their case against the defendant.

Elements of a crime

In order for a crime to be committed, the prosecution must prove the elements of a crime; that is the 'mens rea' and 'actus reus'.

The mens rea is Latin for 'guilty mind'. It is the intention to bring about a particular consequence. This includes an active intention and also recklessness.

The actus reus is Latin for 'guilty act'. It is the physical act.

EXAMPLE OF ELEMENTS OF A CRIME

A health professional is found with medication in her handbag that has come from the hospital. In order for a prosecution of theft to be proved the prosecution will have to establish the *mens rea*, the guilty mind. The health professional must be aware at the time of the crime that they intended to steal the medication.

The prosecution must also prove the *actus reus*, that is, the medication was physically taken by the health professional.

If there was no requirement for the mens rea to be present then the health professional could be convicted of theft in a situation where the medication is accidentally dropped into her handbag and then inadvertently taken home.

An example of a criminal case where a health professional was convicted is the case of GP Harold Shipman. By virtue of its seriousness, this case also culminated in a public inquiry.

REFERENCES

1 Coroners Act 1988 section 1(1)(a).
2 Nursing and Midwifery Council. *Confirmation of Death by Registered Nurses*. London:

NMC; 2008. Available at: www.nmc-uk.org/aDisplayDocument.aspx?documentID=4020 (accessed 20 April 2009).

3 The retention and use of human tissue is governed by the Human Tissue Act 2004.

4 R (on the application of Touche) v HM Coroner for Inner North London district 2001 EWCA Civ 383; 2001 QB 1206 CA.

5 Coroners Act 1988 section 1(1)(a).

6 Coroners Act 1988 section 11(6).

7 Coroners Act 1988 section 11(2).

8 R v Beverly Allitt 1992 [2007] EWHC 2845 (QB).

9 R v Harold Shipman 2000. www.the-shipman-inquiry.org.uk/trialday.asp?Day=58 (accessed 3 April 2009).

10 *Male nurse used sedative to kill and rape*; www.guardian.co.uk/Archive/Article/0,4273, 4019340,00.html (accessed 3 April 2009).

11 R v Adomako (1995) 1 AC 171; 1994 3 All ER 79 1 AC 171.

12 R v Beverly Allitt 1992, op. cit.

13 Police and Criminal Evidence Act 1984 (PACE).

CHAPTER 5

The case of Harold Shipman*

On Monday, 31 January 2000 the jury at Preston Crown Court convicted GP Harold Shipman of 15 murders and of forging a Will.

Kathleen Grundy, an 81-year-old widow, ex-Mayoress of Hyde, was a patient of the GP whom she respected and trusted. She had followed him when he set up his solo practice and shortly before her death had even considered making a £200 donation to his practice fund. She was found dead on 24 June 1998 after she failed to arrive at the Age Concern Club where she helped serve meals for other pensioners.

Mrs Grundy's daughter, Angela Woodruff, a solicitor, was told of her mother's death in a phone call from the police. She called the surgery where Shipman's wife, Primrose, answered the phone and took a message. When Shipman called back, he told Mrs Woodruff a post-mortem was not necessary because he had seen her so soon before her death.

Mrs Woodruff's suspicions were not aroused until a few days later when she was contacted by the Hamilton Ward legal firm handling her mother's Will. Her own law practice in Warwick, which specialised in probate, had usually dealt with her mother's legal affairs. The original Will had been lodged with the firm in 1986. Hamilton Ward had received a new Will the same day that Mrs Grundy died. The new Will was badly typed.

Mrs Woodruff told the Shipman trial in October:

---

* The text of this chapter has been previously published and is reproduced here with the kind permission of the original author, Gerald England. England G. *An Account of the Murderous GP of Hyde*. Available at: www.geraldengland.co.uk/gx/shipman.htm (accessed 30 April 2009).

> My mother was a meticulously tidy person. The thought of her signing a docu-
> ment which is so badly typed didn't make any sense. The signature looked
> strange, it looked too big. The concept of Mum signing a document leaving
> everything to her doctor was unbelievable.

The Will also failed to mention a second house that her mother owned.
Mrs Woodruff contacted the police after speaking to the two witnesses she
believed to have signed the document.

The police exhumed Mrs Grundy's body and found traces of morphine.
They also recovered the Brother typewriter used for writing the Will from
Shipman's surgery. Shipman told Mrs Woodruff, and maintained in court,
that Mrs Grundy had been suffering chest pains shortly before her death. Mrs
Woodruff, however, said that she had spoken to her mother a few days earlier
and found her as lively as ever. She had been looking forward to a weekend
outing to Derbyshire, she told the court. Shipman visited Mrs Grundy at
home on the morning of 24 June, ostensibly to take a blood sample. It was
then that he injected her with a lethal dose of diamorphine. To cover his
tracks Shipman had changed Mrs Grundy's records to make a false medical
history.

Shipman was born in Nottingham on 14 January 1946. When he was 17
his mother, Vera, died of lung cancer at the age of 43. In 1965 he went to
study medicine at Leeds University. In 1970, Shipman graduated from university and started working at the Pontefract General Infirmary. By 1974 he
had become a GP working in a practice in Todmorden, but he soon began
to have blackouts.

At first it was thought he had epilepsy, but it turned out that he was
addicted to the morphine-like drug pethidine. He was fired from his job at
the Todmorden practice. Shipman admitted to charges of making out drug
prescriptions to himself, forgery and fraud. His only explanation was that
he had become fascinated with drugs while at college. He was convicted at
Halifax Magistrates Court in February 1976 and fined £600.

The senior partner at the Todmorden practice, Dr Michael Grieve, said:

> If [Shipman] hadn't at that point gone straight into hospital, perhaps his sen-
> tence would have been more than just a fine. I think it's perhaps the fact that
> he put his hand up and said 'I need treatment' and went into hospital, and then
> the sick-doctor routine takes over.

The GMC at the time did not see fit to strike him off.

Although he was barred from taking any job that gave him access to drugs, he managed to find work as a clinical medical officer at Bishop Auckland Hospital. In 1977, Shipman re-emerged as a GP in Hyde. His new colleagues at the Donnybrook Surgery respected his work, although some felt he could be arrogant and patronising towards his patients, but his patients loved his friendly bedside manner. He supported local schools and the St John's Ambulance Brigade and was regarded as a pillar of society. In 1992, he split from the Donnybrook practice to set up on his own, around the corner in Market Street. It is rumoured that he left behind a massive unpaid tax bill, but took with him a very large list of patients. His wife, Primrose, worked as a part-time receptionist.

Suspicions about him started to emerge in 1997. Staff at Massey's undertakers had begun to notice that they were performing a lot of funerals where the deceased were older ladies who lived alone, were not noticeably ill previously and had been found dead either by Dr Shipman himself or shortly after he had visited them. At the same time doctors at the Brooke Surgery, a joint practice across the road from Shipman's surgery, were also concerned about the number of deaths at his surgery, compared to the number of deaths at their own surgery. These concerns were passed via the local coroner to the police. However, as there was no firm evidence to back up these suspicions, the police were unable to question Shipman about them.

Angela Woodruff did her own detective work to determine that her mother's new Will was forged. Armed with this evidence, the police were able to arrest Shipman on suspicion of fraud and question him. The police exhumed a number of bodies from Hyde Cemetery. In the end Shipman was charged with a total of 15 murders.

The earliest murder of which Shipman was convicted occurred on 6 March 1995. Marie West was injected with diamorphine whilst her friend waited in the kitchen. Shipman claimed she had died of a massive stroke. Police found her medical records at the doctor's home.

Irene Turner had recently returned from holiday with a cold when she was visited at home by Shipman on 11 July 1996. The doctor killed her with a morphine injection. As she lay dying, Shipman told a neighbour to pack clothes for Mrs Turner as she needed to go to hospital. No ambulance came and Shipman claimed she had died from diabetes.

When Harold Shipman was discovered in the home of Lizzie Adams by one of her friends on 28 February 1997, he claimed he had phoned for an ambulance then pretended to cancel it when it was clear the 77-year-old dancing teacher was dead. Phone records show no such calls were made. Shipman said she died of pneumonia. Her medical records were found in a carrier bag in his garage.

On 25 April 1997 Shipman called on Jean Lilley. A neighbour saw him leave and went to see her friend, but found her dead. Shipman said the 59-year-old had died of heart failure. A pathologist found no evidence of severe heart problems and found cause of death to be morphine poisoning.

Dr Shipman killed Ivy Lomas, 63, at his surgery on 29 May 1997. He then saw three other patients before telling anyone she had died. He also altered her medical records two days later. Shipman told police and his receptionist conflicting stories of how she had died. The court heard how the GP had considered Mrs Lomas a 'nuisance', because she was such a regular attendee at the surgery.

Muriel Grimshaw was found dead in her home on 14 July 1997 by her daughter. Shipman claimed she had died from a stroke and hypertension. He then altered her medical records to hide her cause of death.

Marie Quinn was killed by an injection of morphine at her home on 24 November 1997. Shipman told her son that she had phoned him saying she thought she'd had a stroke. The doctor said she was dead by the time he arrived at her home. Phone records show no such call was made, nor was there any evidence that Mrs Quinn had suffered from the problems he said she had.

Kathleen Wagstaff died on 9 December 1997. Shipman claimed he had received a call to attend Mrs Wagstaff, but records show no such call was made. He also said her death was due to heart disease, but no evidence was found.

Bianka Pomfret phoned Shipman for a home visit on 10 December 1997 and was later found dead in her chair. Shipman claimed she had heart trouble and had died of coronary thrombosis and ischaemic heart disease. Experts found Shipman had altered Mrs Pomfret's records in the hour before her body was discovered to generate a backdated history of heart disease.

Norah Nuttall was visited at her home on 26 January 1998. Less than an hour later her son returned to find his mother slumped in a chair. Dr Shipman said he had called an ambulance; when Mrs Nuttall was found to be dead he pretended to make another call to cancel it. Phone records showed the GP had neither ordered nor cancelled an ambulance.

Pamela Hillier was an active 68-year-old who had been stripping wallpaper the week before her death. She was found dead on 9 February 1998, by paramedics who said the police should be told. Dr Shipman said she had died of a massive stroke and there was no need for a post-mortem. Police computer experts found he had made 10 changes to her medical records in the two hours before her body was found, to support his diagnosis.

Maureen Ward, 57, had been suffering from cancer, but was not in ill health at the time of her death on 18 February 1998. Shipman reported her death to the warden at the flats where she lived, saying the cause was a brain tumour. Shipman murdered her using diamorphine, before reporting that her sudden death had been caused by a brain tumour. He then altered her medical records to suggest her cancer had spread to her brain. A cancer specialist who had seen her a month earlier told the court there were no signs that her cancer had returned.

Winifred Mellor, 73, was found dead in her chair on 11 May 1998, having been complaining of a sinus problem. Shipman was reported to have visited her earlier in the day. After a cursory examination, he claimed she had died of coronary thrombosis – despite the fact she was fit enough to go on a two-hour walk only weeks before her death. Shipman altered her medical records to make it look like she had complained to him of chest pains.

Joan Melia, 73, visited Shipman at his surgery on 12 June 1998, suffering from a chest infection. He made a house call to her the same day and she was later found dead in her chair. The GP did not bother to examine her before issuing a death certificate for pneumonia aggravated by emphysema. A pathologist later found evidence of morphine, but not of serious lung problems.

Kathleen Grundy was the last of his victims to die. She was in good health and very active the day before her death on 24 June 1998. She was visited by Shipman early that morning for a blood sample and was later found dead, sitting on her settee. When her body was exhumed one month later, high amounts of morphine were found. There was no record of any blood sample having been taken and Shipman also falsified written and computer records to make it look as though Mrs Grundy was a drug abuser.

The Harold Fred Shipman case is unusual. This was not the culmination of police enquiries into unsolved murders. Until Shipman was arrested, few suspected that any murders had taken place. Although many of the relatives and friends of these victims were unhappy about the way Dr Shipman had treated these women, until he forged Kathleen Grundy's Will, they did not know about how others had died in similar circumstances. There was no one to compare notes with. Even when the undertakers and other doctors noticed an anomalous number of deaths, because Shipman had forged medical records there was no evidence to warrant a more thorough investigation. Once the facts were known, many more put two and two together about events surrounding the deaths of their own relatives. Police considered further charges.

It was reported early in 2000 that the police were investigating 192 deaths. Although they had enough evidence to prosecute in at least 23 cases, it was decided not to prosecute. The decision was made on the basis that due to the publicity surrounding the original prosecution and convictions for the first 15 cases, a *fair trial* would not be possible. Whilst some relatives were OK with the decision – you can't hang a dog twice – others were angry and called for a full public inquiry. (Public inquiry is discussed in Chapter 7.)

Inquests into the deaths of former patients started in August 2000. On 16 August 2000, the coroner's verdict was that Sarah Ashworth had been unlawfully killed. The same verdict was given following the inquests on Alice Kitchen and Elizabeth Mellor.

More inquests took place in 2001. In the first case of an inquest on someone who had been cremated, Hilda Hibbert, the coroner ruled that she had been unlawfully killed. Although forensic evidence wasn't available, the circumstantial evidence was so strong that no other verdict was deemed possible.

By April 2001 a total of 27 inquests had taken place. Only in two cases was an open verdict given – the coroner deciding that there was insufficient evidence to reach a verdict of unlawful killing.

The police had a list of a further 299 patients whom they believed may have been killed by Shipman. The Home Office has yet to decide whether there will be further inquests in these cases.

Meanwhile, moves were afoot to have the surgery from which he operated moved to new premises. Many of Shipman's former patients would have liked to stay with Dr Haz Lloyd, the locum who had been caring for them since Shipman's arrest. However, West Pennine Health Authority said they could only hand the practice over to a local doctor who was on their list of principal GPs.

West Pennine Health Authority transferred the 2800-patient list to the practice led by Dr Amy Cumming. From 3 October 2000, the patients came under the care of GP Lisa Gutteridge, based at the surgery in Great Norbury Street. Dr Haz Lloyd has not joined that practice. The move was opposed by the 21 Market Street Action Group – a group of former Shipman patients loyal to Dr Lloyd.

In January 2001, the Department of Health published a report by Professor Richard Baker. He had undertaken a clinical review of deaths under Dr Shipman from 1974 when he was practicing in Todmorden until 1998 when he was at the Donneybrook practice. The report reveals that there were almost 300 more deaths among his patients than among those of other doctors. Clusters of deaths being reported in the early afternoon, occurring unexpectedly to mainly elderly women patients, suggests that many of these were probably the result of murderous intervention on the part of the doctor. It is also clear that his killing spree did not start when he opened up his one-man practice on Market Street, but that he had been murdering patients at the practice in Todmorden and whilst a member of the Donneybrook team.

As a result of the report, the police added 62 cases to the number under active investigation.

West Yorkshire police investigated all the 22 deaths which occurred in Todmorden during Shipman's time there.

Estimates of the number of people killed by Shipman ranged from a conservative 76 to over 1000.

On 13 January 2004, Shipman hanged himself in his cell at Wakefield Jail. He never broke his silence about why he committed so many murders.[1,2]

REFERENCES

1 England G. *An Account of the Murderous GP of Hyde*. Available at: www.geraldengland. co.uk/gx/shipman.htm (accessed 30 April 2009).
2 The Victim Support Services in Tameside have a website: www.victimsupport-tameside. co.uk

CHAPTER 6

Manslaughter, gross negligence and recklessness

Of course such cases involving deliberate harm are a rare occurrence. In the usual course of events the health professional does not intend to cause deliberate harm.

The health professional in the context of clinical responsibility will be concerned with how criminal liability might arise in the normal course of their duty. An example is where a patient dies as a result of treatment that was grossly negligent; this can constitute the common law offence of manslaughter. The case of R v Adomako is an illustration of this.[1]

R v ADOMAKO 1994

This case involved manslaughter by an anaesthetist when, during surgery, the endotracheal tube disconnected and this went unnoticed by the anaesthetist. The supply of oxygen to the patient ceased, which led to cardiac arrest and death.

The anaesthetist first became aware that something was wrong when the alarm sounded on the Dinamap machine, which monitors the patient's blood pressure. The evidence was that almost five minutes had elapsed between the disconnection and the alarm sounding. Following the alarm, the anaesthetist responded in various ways by checking the equipment and administering atropine to raise the patient's blood pressure. But at no stage before the cardiac

> arrest did the anaesthetist check the endotracheal tube connection. The disconnection was not discovered until after resuscitation measures had been commenced.

This was considered to be so reckless and grossly negligent that it constituted manslaughter.

The courts directed in this case that in order to establish manslaughter by gross negligence the ordinary principles of the law of negligence applied to ascertain whether the defendant had been in breach of duty to the person who had died. If so, the jury must go on to consider whether that breach of duty should be characterised as gross negligence and therefore as a crime.

> That would depend on the seriousness of the breach and the extent to which the defendant's conduct departed from the proper standard of care incumbent upon him, involving as it must have done, a risk of death to the patient, was such that it should be judged criminal.[2]

A health professional may commit a criminal offence of assault and battery, where, for example, he treats a patient without valid consent.

EXAMPLE OF ASSAULT AND BATTERY

A mother with her son of eight years and daughter of seven years attended the dentist. An appointment had been made only for the mother and daughter. Whilst in the waiting room the son went to the bathroom. He was missing for about 15 minutes when his mother became worried. She went to look for him and found him in the dentist chair. Her son had been seen in the corridor by the dentist who said, 'Come on chappy, in the chair.' The dentist then proceeded to give him the treatment that was intended for the daughter. The dentist extracted two second healthy molars.

This constitutes not only a breach of duty of care giving rise to a civil claim for damages, but also a criminal offence of assault and battery, as there was no consent to treat the patient.

Other areas where criminal charges may also be brought is where there is a case of fraud or theft.

DEFENCES TO A CRIMINAL CHARGE

There are a number of main defences to a criminal charge that may affect health professionals.

The absence of *mens rea* or *actus reus*

This is the absence of the guilty mind or guilty act. This could be, for example, the unintentional taking of the medication that had accidentally fallen into the health professional's handbag. There would be no guilty mind, as the health professional did not deliberately intend to steal the medication.

Insanity

At the time the offence was committed the accused was insane. The definition of insanity as a defence is laid down by the McNaughten Rules 1843.[3]

- That every man is sane and possesses a sufficient degree of reason to be responsible for his crimes, until the contrary can be proved.
- To establish a defence on the grounds of insanity, it must be proved that at the time of committing the act, the person was labouring under such a defect of reason, from disease of the mind, as to not know the nature of the act he was doing, or if he did know, he did not know what he was doing was wrong.

Diminished responsibility

The Homicide Act 1957[4] introduced 'diminished responsibility' as a defence in cases of unlawful killing, which would normally invoke the mandatory life sentence for murder (at the time there was also the death penalty). It only applies to the offence of unlawful killing. It allows for a defendant to be convicted of manslaughter instead of murder by virtue of his diminished responsibility.

> If he was suffering from such abnormality of mind (whether arising from a condition of arrested or retarded development of mind or any inherent causes or reduced by disease or injury) as substantially impaired his mental responsibility for his acts and omissions in doing or being the party to the killing.[5]

Mistake

There is a general rule that ignorance of the criminal law is no defence, even if the ignorance is reasonable in the circumstances. However, a mistake of fact may provide a defence to a criminal charge as the accused may not have the necessary *mens rea* required to prove the criminal offence. For example, a mistaken fact is that a person was present at the material time when in fact they were not.

Necessity

Necessity arises where a defendant is forced by circumstances to disobey the criminal law. Although there are incidences where it has been accepted as a defence to murder, for example in the case of R v Bourne,[6] the generally accepted position is that necessity cannot be a defence to a criminal charge.

R v BOURNE 1939

In the case of R v Bourne the defendant gynaecologist performed an abortion on a young girl who had been raped. He had formed the opinion that she could die if permitted to give birth, and the operation was performed in a public hospital, with the consent of her parents. The defendant was found not guilty of 'unlawfully procuring a miscarriage' following a direction from the trial judge to the jury that a defendant did not act 'unlawfully' for the purposes of section 58 Offences Against the Person Act 1861,[7] where he acted in good faith, in the exercise of his clinical judgement. (This is now within the Abortion Act 1967.[8])

Duress or coercion

Duress or coercion may be a valid defence to a crime if it can be established that the force or compulsion was such that the accused has no choice, usually in circumstances where there is a fear of death or serious bodily injury.

Superior orders

It is not a defence for the accused to argue that the crime was committed because they were obeying orders of their superior (known as the Nuremberg Defence). It might, however, be possible for the health professional to show that as a result of the orders they lacked the *mens rea* of the crime and that they were acting reasonably in the circumstances.

Following orders in relation to other areas of accountability is considered later in Chapter 11.

Self-defence

A person may defend themselves or defend another person against an attack, or defend their property, provided they use reasonable force. If the force is not reasonable they could find themselves liable to prosecution for assault, murder or manslaughter.

In common law the defence of self-defence operates in three ways. It allows a person to use reasonable force to:

➤ defend himself from an attack
➤ prevent an attack on another person, for example R v Rose 1884,[9] where the defendant who had shot dead his father whilst the latter was launching a murderous attack on the defendant's mother, was acquitted of murder on the grounds of self-defence
➤ defend his property.

In addition, section 3(1) of the Criminal Law Act 1967[10] provides that:

> A person may use such force as is reasonable in the circumstances in the prevention of crime, or in effecting or assisting in the lawful arrest of offenders or suspected offenders or of persons unlawfully at large.

Both the common law and statutory defences can be raised in respect of any crime with which the defendant is charged, and if successful will result in the defendant being completely acquitted. However, if a defendant uses excessive force this indicates that he acted unreasonably in the circumstances. There will be no valid defence, and the defendant will be found guilty of the crime.

CORPORATE MANSLAUGHTER AND CORPORATE HOMICIDE ACT 2007

The aim of the Act

The aim of the Corporate Manslaughter and Corporate Homicide Act 2007[11] is to set out more clearly the extent of the duty of care owed by companies and other organisations and to overcome some of the legal technicalities, which, in the past, have made it difficult to secure successful convictions of corporate defendants. The offence is aimed at cases where management failures lie across an organisation. It is the organisation itself that will face prosecution.

In England, Wales and Northern Ireland, the new offence will be called corporate manslaughter. In Scotland it will be called corporate homicide. The Act came into force on 6 April 2008. Under the Act it is now a criminal offence whereby an organisation manages or organises its activities in a way that causes a person's death,[12] and amounts to a gross breach of a relevant duty of care owed by the organisation to the deceased.[13]

How is a gross duty of care determined?

A breach of duty will be gross if the conduct of the organisation falls far below what can reasonably be expected of the organisation in the circumstances. Ultimately that will be a matter of fact for a jury to decide.

How does the duty of care arise?

The duty of care can arise in a number of ways. The following duties fall within the ambit of the Act:
> a duty owed to employees or others working for the organisation
> a duty owed as an occupier of premises
> a duty arising from the supply of goods or services (which includes healthcare services)
> a duty arising from the carrying out of construction or maintenance
> a duty arising from the use or keeping of any plant or vehicle.

Who does the Act apply to?

The Act applies to corporations, police forces, partnerships and organisations as set out in a schedule. 'Organisations' includes all the major government departments, such as the Department of Health. The Act therefore applies to all NHS bodies.[14] It also applies to corporations registered as operating a care home or any other care establishment or agency. It will also apply to partnerships operating such establishments or agencies.

The Act specifically extends the duties of care caught by the Act to include duties owed to persons whose safety is the responsibility of the organisation. This provision was introduced to bring deaths in custody within the ambit of the Act. Persons affected include:
> a person detained in a custodial institution or in a custody area at a court or police station
> a person detained at a removal centre or a short-term holding facility
> a person being transported in a vehicle, or being held in the course of a prison escort or immigration escort

➤ a person living in secure accommodation
➤ a person who is a detained patient.

The Act will therefore impact heavily on NHS bodies providing healthcare to patients detained either under the Mental Health Act 1983[15] or within prisons.

The NHS, duty of care and public policy decisions

The application of the Act is limited when an organisation is carrying out 'exclusively public functions'. An NHS body predominantly carries out 'exclusively public functions'. Therefore, where an NHS body is carrying out such functions, its activities will be caught by the Act only in specific circumstances.

Those circumstances include:
➤ where the duty of care is owed to an employee or other person working for the organisation
➤ where the duty of care arises out of the NHS body's occupation of premises; or
➤ where the duty of care is owed to a detained patient or a person living in secure accommodation.

If it can be established that an NHS body is carrying out functions that are not exclusively public, for example, then the above limitation to the potential criminal liability under the Act will not apply. For example, where a Foundation Trust operates a private clinic, the Act will apply without the above limitation.

However, even in those circumstances where the Act does not apply, an NHS body can still be prosecuted for breaches of the substantive health and safety legislation in the provision of healthcare to patients, as happened in the well publicised prosecution of Southampton University Hospitals NHS Trust.[16]

Any duty of care, which an organisation might owe arising from deciding matters of public policy, will not be caught by the Act. This would exclude from the ambit of the Act, for example, decisions made by a public body not to licence a new medicine or by a Primary Care Trust (PCT) not to allocate healthcare resources in a particular way.

A public authority, such as the Commission for Social Care Inspection or the Healthcare Commission, will not be criminally liable under the Act in respect of inspections carried out in accordance with its statutory duties, except where there is a gross breach of the duty of care owed to its employees or of its duty of care as an occupier.

The duty of care and emergencies – the exemption

Any duty of care owed by an NHS body in respect of the way in which it responds to emergency circumstances will not fall within the Act, except where the duty is owed to employees or as an occupier of premises. Organisations with emergency responsibilities are listed in the Act and include the providers of the transportation of organs and blood, NHS Trusts and ambulance services.

Emergency is defined within the Act as circumstances that are present and imminent and cause, or are likely to cause, serious harm or worsening of harm. Harm includes serious injury, serious illness, mental illness, harm to plants or animals and harm to property. Clearly this will apply to many of the functions of NHS bodies in the provision of healthcare.

It is important to note, however, that the Act specifically states that the carrying out of medical treatment in an emergency does give rise to a relevant duty caught by the Act, but decisions as to the order in which persons are to be treated do not.

However, if an NHS body can establish that the provision of that emergency medical treatment was carried out whilst the NHS body was fulfilling exclusively public functions, it will not be caught under the Act, except, as stated above, in the situations where the duty of care is owed to employees or other workers, as an occupier, or to detained persons.

The emphasis on senior management responsibility

In order to convict an organisation for corporate manslaughter, it will no longer be necessary for an offence to be proved against an individual within that organisation (the so-called 'controlling mind'). However, the Act makes it clear that an organisation can be convicted for corporate manslaughter only if the way in which its activities are managed or organised by senior managers is a substantial element in the breach of the duty of care.

Senior management means persons who play a significant role in the making of decisions about how the whole or a substantial part of the organisation's activities are to be managed. This includes both centralised, headquarters functions as well as those in operational management roles.

The importance of a health and safety culture

Under a new approach, courts will look at management systems and practices across the organisation, providing a more effective means for prosecuting the worst organisational failures to manage health and safety properly.

A trial jury considering an offence of corporate manslaughter may be invited by the judge to consider the extent to which evidence shows that there were attitudes, policies, systems or accepted practices within the organisation that were likely to have encouraged a failure of the health and safety system or to have produced a tolerance of it.

Managing risks

This is an opportunity for employers to think again about how risks are managed. Organisations should ensure they are taking proper steps to meet current legal duties.

Since 6 April 2008, the Act means that those who disregard the safety of others at work, with fatal consequences, are more vulnerable to very serious criminal charges.

Penalties

An organisation convicted of corporate manslaughter will face an unlimited fine. The Act also provides for courts to impose a publicity order, requiring the organisation to publicise details of its conviction and fine.

No individual can be prosecuted under the Act and, hence, the court cannot impose a custodial sentence. However, individuals who commit a serious breach of a duty of care leading to a person's death may still face prosecution and possible imprisonment for the common law offence of gross negligence manslaughter. The common law offence has been abolished in relation to companies.

Courts may also require an organisation to take steps to address the failures behind the death (a remedial order).

It is the organisation itself which will face prosecution not the senior managers. Individuals can already be prosecuted for gross negligence manslaughter/culpable homicide and for health and safety offences. The Act does not change this and prosecutions against individuals will continue to be taken where there is sufficient evidence and it is in the public interest to do so.

REFERENCES

1 R v Adomako 1995 1 AC 171; 1994 3 All ER 79.
2 Ibid.
3 R v McNaughten 1843 4 St Tr NS 847.
4 Homicide Act 1957 s2.
5 Homicide Act 1957 s2(1).
6 R v Bourne 1939 1 KB 687; 1938 3 All ER 615.
7 Offences Against the Person Act 1861 s58.
8 Abortion Act 1967.
9 R v Rose 1884 15 Cox 540.
10 Criminal Law Act 1967 s3(1).
11 Corporate Manslaughter and Corporate Homicide Act 2007.
12 Corporate Manslaughter and Corporate Homicide Act 2007 s1(1)(a).
13 Corporate Manslaughter and Corporate Homicide Act 2007 s1(1)(b).
14 Corporate Manslaughter and Corporate Homicide Act 2007 Schedule 1.
15 Mental Health Act 1983.
16 Dyer C. Hospital trust prosecuted for not supervising junior doctors. *BMJ*. 2006; **332**: 135.

CHAPTER 7

Civil courts

The civil courts deal with civil matters. This can involve money matters, contractual disputes or property issues. They include negligence, trespass to property or the person, nuisance or breach of statutory duty, amongst other things.

In respect of health professionals, the civil actions that will generally concern them include:

➤ negligence (clinical negligence)
➤ trespass to property or the person
➤ breach of statutory duty.

Where there has been a breach of the civil law then it may give rise to a claim for compensation by the injured party.

For health professionals they are likely to become involved in the civil process where a patient has been injured as a result of the treatment they have received and the patient sues for compensation (damages).

COUNTY COURT AND HIGH COURT

The civil courts in England and Wales are divided into the County Court and the High Court.

The majority of civil cases are heard in the County Court. There are around 218 county courts throughout England and Wales. The High Court sits at the Royal Courts of Justice in London, with satellites as well as some major court centres around the country in major cities and towns (known as the District Registries).

Whether a case is heard in the County Court or the High Court depends on the value of the claim. Currently if a claim is worth over £50 000 it will be heard in the High Court. However, clinical negligence cases can be complex and they are often transferred to the High Court because of their complexities, even though the value may be less than £50 000.

A decision of the County Court may be appealed and will be heard by the High Court. Any subsequent appeal will be heard by the Court of Appeal and then by the House of Lords.

STANDARD OF PROOF

In the civil courts, the standard of proof is 'on the balance of probability'. The court will ask, 'is it more likely than not that a certain set of circumstances occurred?'

In civil cases, it is for the claimant (the party bringing the claim) to prove their case. The term claimant is quite new. Prior to 1999, persons who brought claims in civil courts were referred to as plaintiffs.

See Figure 7.1 for the Civic Court structure.

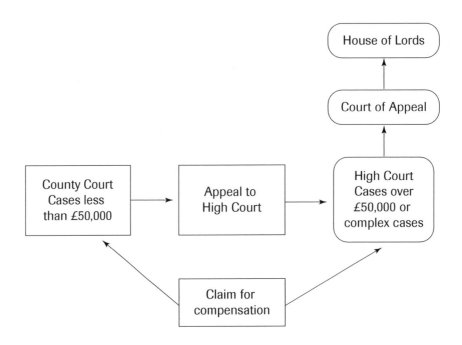

FIGURE 7.1 Simplified version of the Civil Court structure

WITNESS

When a case comes before the civil courts, those health professionals involved in the care of a patient are likely to have to give evidence. They will be required to give an account of the facts surrounding the issues. Although the health professional is accountable to a patient if something were to go wrong, when giving evidence in the civil court the purpose is to establish, for example, whether there has been a breach of duty of care, and whether the patient is entitled to compensation. In this context the health professional in the civil court process is not on trial, although when in the witness box they may feel as if they are!

Remember the purpose of the court process is to obtain the factual information so that the judge or adjudicator can reach a decision. However, the judge may, in hearing the facts during the trial, report a health professional to their professional body.

The components of a civil claim are discussed later in Chapter 8.

PUBLIC INQUIRY

A public inquiry is a formal procedure ordered by the government to investigate matters of public concern.

Typical events for a public inquiry include investigating serious allegations of improper conduct in public service, such as an inquiry into medical misconduct. An example of this was the case of GP, Harold Shipman.[1]

A public inquiry is held in a public environment, which allows interested members of the public and organisations to present their cases orally or via written evidence. A public inquiry is chaired by an official appointed by the government. This could be a judge, an inspector or a member of the civil service.

It is up to the government to decide whether to have a public inquiry. But it can come about if there is pressure put on the government by the public, pressure groups, campaign groups or opposition parties.

THE SHIPMAN INQUIRY

Harold Shipman was convicted of the murder of 15 of his patients, but he was suspected of having murdered many more. Although there was enough evidence to prosecute in at least 23 cases, it was decided not to on the basis that, due to the publicity surrounding the original prosecution and convictions for the first 15 cases, a *fair trial* would not be possible. Relatives of the victims suspected of having been murdered were angry and called for a full public inquiry.

Initially it was announced that an inquiry would be sitting in private, but an appeal to have the inquiry made public was successful. The inquiry was to be held under the auspices of the 1912 Tribunal of Inquiry (Evidence) Act.[2] The previous inquiry held was the Dunblane inquiry in 1996.

In January 2001, it was annnounced that the High Court Judge, Dame Janet Smith would chair the inquiry.

Reports of Dame Janet Smith

At the conclusion of the inquiry, Dame Janet Smith produced a series of reports on several issues each containing a variety of recommendations.

First report

'Death disguised' published 19 July 2002

In the inquiry's first report, the chairman considered how many patients Shipman killed, the means employed and the period of time over which the killings took place.

Second report

The police investigation of March 1998, published 14 July 2003

In the inquiry's second report, the chairman examined the conduct of the police investigation into Shipman that took place in March 1998 and failed to uncover his crimes.

Third report

Death certification and the investigation of deaths by coroners, published 14 July 2003

In the inquiry's third report, the chairman considered the present system for death and cremation certification and for the investigation of deaths by coroners, together with the conduct of those who had operated those systems in the aftermath of the deaths of Shipman's victims. She has made recommendations for change based on her findings.

Fourth report

The regulation of controlled drugs in the community, published 15 July 2004

In the inquiry's fourth report, the chairman considered the systems for the management and regulation of controlled drugs, together with the conduct of those who operated those systems. She has made recommendations for change based upon her findings.

Fifth report

Safeguarding patients: lessons from the past – proposals for the future, published 19 December 2004
In the inquiry's fifth report, the Chairman considered the handling of complaints against GPs, the raising of concerns about GPs, GMC procedures and its proposal for revalidation of doctors. She has made recommendations for change based upon her findings.

Sixth report

Shipman: the final report, published 27 January 2005
In the inquiry's sixth and final report, the Chairman considered how many patients Shipman killed during his career as a junior doctor at Pontefract General Infirmary between 1970 and 1974. She also considered a small number of cases from Shipman's time in Hyde, which the inquiry became aware of after the publication of the first report. Claims by a former inmate at HMP Preston regarding alleged claims by Shipman about the number of patients he had killed were also considered.

The Shipman Inquiry published its final report on 27 January 2005 and was decommissioned in spring 2005.

In response to these reports, the Department of Health published guidelines[3], and policies were implemented.

EMPLOYMENT TRIBUNAL

As discussed in the previous chapter on accountability, the health professional is accountable to their employer. The employer may invoke sanctions, such as being disciplined or even dismissed. If the health professional (employee) considers that, for example, the dismissal was unfair then they may wish to challenge this though the court process.

Bodies known as 'employment tribunals' deal with most work-related legal action. Until 1998 these were known as 'industrial tribunals' having been set up by the Industrial Tribunals Act in 1972.[4] Employment tribunals operate in England, Wales and Scotland. In Northern Ireland the system is similar but the tribunals are called 'fair employment tribunals'.

These tribunals are specialist employment 'courts'. A tribunal will be made up of three people. The chair will be legally qualified, and there will be two lay members – one of whom will be an employee representative and the other will be an employer representative.

Tribunals were originally intended to provide a relatively cheap, speedy and informal means of settling employment rights disputes between employees and employers. While they are still less formal than civil courts they have become more legalistic and formal as employment law has become more complex and specialised. A tribunal will settle disputes about, for example, the contract of employment, whether there has been an unfair dismissal or sexual discrimination. The tribunal may award compensation or make an order to reinstate the employee.

However most claims at tribunals relate to unfair dismissal. Argument is therefore normally about the facts of the matter, rather than legal points.

A health professional who becomes involved in this process may be able to obtain advice from their indemnity insurer.

REFERENCES

1 Harold Shipman Public Inquiry. www.the-shipman-inquiry.org.uk (accessed 20 April 2009).
2 Tribunal of Inquiry (Evidence) Act 1912.
3 Department of Health. *Safeguarding Patients*. London: DoH; 2007. www.dh.gov.uk/en/ Publicationsandstatistics/Publications/PublicationsPolicyAndGuidance/DH_065953 (accessed 20 April 2009).
4 Industrial Tribunals Act 1972.

CHAPTER 8

Civil law and negligence

As discussed in the previous chapter, the civil courts deal with matters of breaches of civil law. Where there has been a breach of the civil law then it may give rise to a claim for compensation by the injured party. Where a patient has been injured as a result of treatment they received then they may be entitled to financial compensation and will pursue their claim through the civil process.

CIVIL PROCEDURE RULES 1998

Matters that go before the civil courts must comply with the Civil Procedure Rules.[1] These rules were implemented in April 1999, following Lord Justice Woolf's report on Access to Justice because the existing system was considered to be too slow, cumbersome and expensive.

The principles behind the Civil Procedure Rules were that litigation should be avoided wherever possible and that court proceedings should be a last resort. Litigation should be less adversarial and more co-operative with the timescales for litigation and bringing the case to trial being shorter.

To assist this process, in clinical negligence claims a pre-action protocol was put in place, namely 'the pre-action protocol in clinical disputes'. This process allows both parties to gather evidence, to share information and to resolve the dispute before considering whether to commence court proceedings. If the matter is not resolved in the pre-action stage then formal proceedings are commenced in the civil courts.

TIME LIMIT

How long after treatment can a patient sue?

The time frame for a person to bring a claim is set out in the Limitation Act 1980.[2] A patient has a certain time limit by which they must commence formal court proceedings. If they do not issue proceedings in court within the time then they will not be able to pursue their claim. They will be 'time barred'.

A patient bringing a claim for compensation for an injury has three years from:

➤ the date on which the cause of action occurred; or
➤ the date of knowledge (if later) of the person injured.

For example:

➤ if a hospital amputates the wrong leg on 2 December 2005 the patient has three years (i.e. until 1 December 2008) to issue a claim in court (i.e. to start proceedings)
➤ a patient has a stomach operation in 1990 and following the operation the patient continues to suffer. On 2 June 2007 the patient undergoes another stomach operation during which the surgeon finds a retained instrument left behind from the operation in 1990. This has been the cause of the patient's ongoing problem. The negligence in leaving the retained instrument occurred in 1990. But the patient's date of knowledge is 2 June 2007 when the instrument was found and when the patient actually became aware of the negligence. So the patient in this case has three years from their date of knowledge (i.e. until 1 June 2010) to issue a claim in court.

Children

A minor, someone under the age of 18 years, has three years from the age of majority (i.e. until they become 21 years of age), or three years from their date of knowledge, to commence their claim in court.

For example:

➤ a child undergoes a tonsillectomy and adenoidectomy at the age of six years. A cleft palate was present at the time and the operation should not have been carried out. The child was left with a speech impediment and suffered both educationally and psychologically. The child has up until they are 21 years of age to bring a claim.

What if the patient dies?

If a person dies before the limitation period expires then the personal representative in the estate can bring a claim within three years of:

➤ the date of death; or
➤ the date of the personal representative's knowledge – whichever is the later.

Discretion of the court

The court has discretion under the Limitation Act 1980 to disregard the time limit. This can be where, for example, someone is under a disability.

For example:

➤ a child suffers permanent brain damage as a result of a delay in delivery at birth. They would be under a mental disability and the court has the discretion to allow the case to proceed even if the time limit has expired. So a child injured at birth could bring a claim when they are, for example, 35 years old.

WHO CAN BRING A CLAIM?

When a patient has been injured as a result of clinical negligence, family members and friends can be angry and upset and may wish to pursue a claim. However, it is not open to all of these people to bring a claim.

The person who has suffered harm as a result of negligent treatment can bring a claim. If that person is a child or is under a mental disability then someone else, for example the person's mother, can bring the claim on their behalf. If there is no suitable person to act on their behalf, the Court of Protection can undertake this task. The Court of Protection can make decisions in relation to the property and affairs and healthcare and personal welfare of adults, and children in certain circumstances, who lack capacity. The Court also has the power to make declarations about whether someone has the capacity to make a particular decision.

If the patient has died as a result of negligence, the executors or personal representatives of the estate of the deceased could bring a claim.

NEGLIGENCE

Health professionals live in fear of being sued. However, it is not as simple as the patient, and sometimes the health professional, would believe. A patient will often demand a particular course of treatment or medication and if they do not get what they want they will threaten to sue. The Trust will sometimes give the patient what they want to avoid being sued. However, in order for a patient to sue there are several legal hurdles that they must overcome. A legal claim cannot be determined simply because there has been an adverse outcome.

Negligence is also referred to as a breach of the duty of care. A breakdown of communication either through system failures or poor records or in some other way may result in injury to the patient. This may give rise to an action in negligence. If a patient is injured as a result of the negligence of a health professional then the patient may sue for financial compensation. (Compensation is also referred to as 'damages'.)

Negligence occurs when the standard of care falls below the reasonable standard expected.

A person who brings a claim for negligence (the person who sues) is called the 'claimant' and the person or organisation being sued is called the 'defendant'. The legal process for bringing a claim is often referred to as 'litigation'.

COMPONENTS OF A LEGAL CLAIM FOR COMPENSATION

Claims for compensations can include:

- ➤ patient falling out of bed
- ➤ pressure sores developing
- ➤ wrong dose of medicine, or at the wrong time, or wrong site
- ➤ wrong limb being amputated
- ➤ treatment given to the wrong patient
- ➤ delay in birth of a baby
- ➤ patient dies as a result of a mistake.

What does the claimant have to show?

TASK

Consider this scenario.

Tom, a keen gardener, also makes homebrew in his garden shed. Having enjoyed a glass of his homebrew he invites his next-door neighbor, Bill, into his garden shed for a tipple of his homebrew.

Bill has a better idea, 'Why don't we go to the pub instead?' Off they go to the pub and they order half a pint of beer each. Tom takes a sip of his beer and says, 'I don't feel very well.' Bill says, 'You look terrible; I think you ought to go to the hospital.'

They arrive at the accident and emergency department and Tom is triaged by the nurse. Tom tells the nurse, 'I had a tipple of my homebrew and then we went to the pub.' The nurse tells Tom, 'You are drunk, go home and sleep it off, if you are not better by the morning go and see your GP.'

By the morning Tom was dead. Tom had inadvertently drunk paraquat in his garden shed. An assumption had been made by the triage nurse that Tom was drunk.

Do you think Tom's family would succeed in claiming compensation?

We will review the answer at the end of the chapter.

In order for a patient to succeed in suing for compensation the onus is upon them to establish the legal principles. They have to establish all of the following:

1 that the defendant owed the claimant a duty of care
2 that the defendant breached that duty of care
3 that such breach 'caused' the injury or loss, known as causation
4 that the injury was 'reasonably foreseeable'
5 and that as a result the claimant has suffered loss.

These principles are explored in more detail later in this chapter.

DUTY OF CARE

Does a health professional owe a duty of care to anyone? To whom do they owe the duty? The patient, the patient's family or the visitor?

Donoghue v Stevenson 1932

The leading case of Donoghue v Stevenson changed the law relating to negligence and is commonly referred to as 'the snail in the ginger beer case'.

A claimant who wishes to bring a claim in negligence has to meet the requirements set out by the House of Lords in this case (Donoghue v Stevenson 1932).[3]

FACTS OF THE CASE

Mrs Donoghue and her friend were out shopping and stopped for refreshments. Mrs Donoghue's friend treated Mrs Donoghue to a bottle of ginger beer. Her friend treated her not only to the ginger beer, but also to a decomposing snail that was lurking in the bottom of the bottle. The experience made Mrs Donoghue sick.

Mrs Donoghue sued the café proprietor. The law at this time was based on contractual obligations. The court said Mrs Donoghue had no contract with the café proprietor; it was her friend who had the contract as it was she who had bought the ginger beer. This was sound legal argument at that time and there was no remedy under the law.

So Mrs Donoghue sued the ginger beer manufacturer. The manufacturer's contract was with the café proprietor, but the manufacturer did not have a contract with Mrs Donoghue and so she lost again.

The matter then went to the Court of Appeal and it was lost on the same principles. There was no contract between Mrs Donoghue, the ginger beer manufacturer or the café proprietor.

Not content with the outcome, Mrs Donoghue took the matter to the House of Lords. What drove her to do that we will never know!

The House of Lords said you must take reasonable care to avoid acts or omissions that you can reasonably foresee would be likely to injure your neighbour.

Your 'neighbour' is considered to be anyone who may be affected by your actions.

The implication of this case is that although there was no contract between Mrs Donoghue and the manufacturer, because Mrs Donoghue was affected by the actions of the manufacturer they must owe her a duty of care.

So the duty of care can be said to exist if your actions are reasonably likely to cause harm to another person.

In this case the court set out three principles that must be present in order for a person to succeed in a claim for compensation for negligence.

In this case the three requirements that the claimant had to show were:
- the defendant **owed** the claimant a duty of care and
- the defendant **breached** that duty of care and
- the defendant's breach of duty **caused** the damage to the claimant.

The court will determine as a matter of course that a Trust or health professional will owe a duty of care to their patient.

TO WHOM DO YOU OWE THE DUTY OF CARE?

The health professional

It follows from the 'neighbour' principle that a health professional will owe a duty of care to their patient. In the course of delivery of care, the health professional's duty is to the patient and not their family. For example, consent to treatment is up to the patient and the family have no right to consent on the patient's behalf. (Consent is a complicated topic and health professionals may wish to read further on this topic in the book entitled Consent in this series.)

However, the health professional will owe a duty to the patient's family and visitors coming onto the premises or, for example, carers in community care.

EXAMPLE OF DUTY OF CARE

If a health visitor rushes upstairs to assist a patient and in doing so knocks over a child who was on the stairs at the time and injures the child, then the health professional will owe the child a duty of care.

The health professional must take reasonable care to avoid acts or omissions that they can reasonably see are likely to cause injury.

Remember the principle of vicarious liability of the employer which was discussed in Chapter 2. Where a patient sues for compensation they will usually sue the Trust rather than the individual.

The Trust

A Trust has a duty of care to ensure the safety of all people, not only patients, in hospitals and in other NHS buildings. A Trust will owe a duty of care to patients, family and visitors on the premises. Where, for example, a visitor dies as a result of a fall on hospital premises the Trust may be faced with a claim for compensation and may also be fined in the criminal courts for breaching health and safety laws. This happened with South West London and St George's Mental Health Trust.[4]

The duty of care owed may be increased towards a person who lacks insight or is more vulnerable.

EXAMPLE OF DUTY OF CARE TO THOSE WHO ARE MORE VULNERABLE

Workmen in a hospital car park digging a large hole placed a notice: 'Beware men at work.'

What about a blind visitor if there is no barrier, just a sign?

A greater duty of care is owed to those who are not sighted. The Trust will have failed in their duty of care.

Public services

A duty of care can also be owed by a public service such as the ambulance service, social services, education, police or fire and rescue service.

KENT v GRIFFITHS 1998

The Court of Appeal held that although the ambulance service owed no duty to the public at large to respond to a telephone call for help, once a 999 call had been accepted the ambulance service had an obligation to provide the service for the named individual at a specified address.[5]

PHELPS v HILLINGDON LONDON BOROUGH COUNCIL 1998

In this case an educational psychologist was employed by the local education authority to give it advice in respect of children in its schools who had learning disabilities. The House of Lords held that a local education authority is liable for the negligent actions of a teacher or educational psychologist and can be sued for a failure to provide an education commensurate with the child's needs.[6]

Reasonable care must be taken to avoid acts or omissions that can be reasonably seen to be likely to cause injury.

WHAT CONSTITUTES A BREACH OF DUTY OF CARE?

'Would a responsible body of medical practitioners have acted in the same way?'

We have established that the health professional owes the patient a duty of care. In order for the patient's claim for compensation to succeed the patient also has to show that the duty of care was breached and that the breach caused the patient harm.

What standard of conduct does the healthcare professional have to reach to fulfil the duty? How do we measure when the duty has been breached?

The test as to whether health professionals are in breach of their duty of care is whether a responsible body of medical practitioners would have acted in the same way. A responsible body is judged on the skill of the health professional. This is known as the 'Bolam principle' and arises from the following case.

BOLAM v FRIERN BARNET 1957

'Where a case involves some special skill or competence then the test as to whether there has been negligence or not is based upon the standard of the ordinary skilled man exercising and professing to have that special skill or knowledge.'[7]

The perceived negligence of a health professional, for example a nurse, will be determined by the standard of the ordinary skilled nurse. This has the effect that the greater the skill, experience and expertise of the health pro-fessional, the greater the duty of care. For example, a specialist nurse, say in diabetes, will owe a greater duty of care than a non-specialist nurse.

The test is a mirror image of you. You will be judged with your knowledge and experience and qualifications and the greater your knowledge, experi-ence and qualifications the greater your duty.

TASK

A doctor makes an error in treating a patient when there is a student present.
What is the duty of the student?

The student may not have the skill, knowledge or expertise to realise that the doctor is making an error. The doctor will be in breach of the duty of care, but the student may not be.

TASK

A doctor makes an error in treating a patient when there is a student nurse.
What is the duty of the staff nurse?

The staff nurse will have greater experience, skill and knowledge than the student and will owe a duty to challenge the doctor's treatment. If the patient suffers as a result of the doctor's treatment the staff nurse will be as liable as the doctor.

EXAMPLE OF LIABILITY

Mr Smith loved his car; he would polish it every day. He took his car out on the road in icy conditions. Mr Jones' car slid into Mr Smith's car on the icy road. In the normal course of events this was an accident. However, Mr Smith pursued a claim against Mr Jones. At trial it was contended that Mr Jones was displaying a badge that said 'institute of advanced motorists'.

If he had been a normal driver Mr Smith would not have brought a claim, but as an advanced driver Mr Jones failed in his duty of care. By his advanced certificate he was holding himself out as possessing greater skills than the normal driver. Therefore he was expected to have been able to avoid the accident. Mr Jones was deemed to be liable for the accident.

During the process of a legal claim a 'letter of claim' is sent to the defendants setting out the details and it will often state 'the care given fell below a reasonable or acceptable standard of care', rather than use the word 'negligent'.

It is for the claimant to prove that the healthcare professional was in breach of his duty of care.

The matter will be judged on what the practice was at the time of the alleged negligence and not what is known subsequently. You cannot judge yesterday's treatment by today's standards.

EXAMPLE OF TIME OF NEGLIGENCE

In the case of haemophiliacs receiving blood, some patients contracted HIV or hepatitis because the blood was not screened. You have to consider whether at the time blood was given there was knowledge of the risks. Now blood is routinely screened, but a patient can only succeed in a claim if the blood was given after the risks were known.

Adverse outcome

A patient cannot sue for compensation simply because there has been an adverse outcome. The question is, how did they arrive at that adverse outcome?

We always hope that a patient benefits from care, but sometimes they do not because there are risks. In the normal course of events a health professional does not deliberately intend to cause harm to a patient. Sometimes the health professional may act in ways that are matters of regret, but they are not necessarily negligent. Sometimes they may be an error of judgement but not negligence.

The court process, by its nature, looks back with the benefit of hindsight. Looking back, the health professional could have made a different decision. But hindsight is a wonderful thing. Had they known what the adverse result would be, of course the health professional would have made a different decision or taken a different course of action. If we could we would never get it wrong, but nobody can predict the outcome. If you make a wrong decision but a responsible choice then there is no negligence.

When a matter goes before the court it is usually the grey areas that are deliberated. Remember the adversarial process: two or more parties with different versions of events. You will say it was an error of judgement but not negligent. The other side will say that it was negligent. You will have to justify your actions and the court, having heard the evidence, has to make a decision on the balance of probabilities.

WHITEHOUSE v JORDAN

A baby was born brain damaged. His mother argued that he was injured because the doctor was 'pulling too long and too strongly' and that the baby should have been born by caesarean section and that had it been, the baby would not have been brain damaged.

The doctor decided to attempt a ventouse delivery first before deciding whether a caesarean section was appropriate. The doctor said he did not know he was going to encounter the difficulties he subsequently encountered.

Some doctors would carry out a caesarean section and some would not.

The doctor said, 'Some might say with hindsight that I made an error of judgement but I was never unprofessional or negligent.'

The judge said an error of clinical judgement is not necessarily negligence.[8]

You cannot establish negligence by outcome if it was an appropriate decision at the time it was made. You cannot say that simply because it went wrong there is a claim.

Whether an error of judgement is a breach of duty of care or not will depend upon the facts of the situation.

EXAMPLE OF DIFFERENT FACTS

A patient may try to sue because they suffered an adverse reaction to medication. If at the time the medication was given there was no reason to suspect that they would suffer such allergic reaction, then in these circumstances there would be no breach of duty of care.

It would be quite a different matter, however, if the patient were given penicillin with a known allergy because the health professional had failed to record the allergy appropriately or failed to read the records before prescribing and administering it.

There are many circumstances which may give rise to a breach of duty of care. Sometimes there are circumstances that may not necessarily be within the control of the health professionals, but nevertheless might give rise to a breach of duty of care, for which the health professional will be accountable. These include:

➤ following approved practice
➤ deviation from approved practice
➤ following policies, protocols, procedures and guidelines
➤ keeping up-to-date
➤ new and developing practices
➤ competency
➤ team decisions
➤ obeying orders
➤ waiting lists
➤ poor communication including poor record-keeping and system failures
➤ delegating
➤ supervising
➤ pressures on managers and staff
➤ risk managing
➤ governance
➤ whistle-blowing.

These are discussed in detail later in Chapter 11.

CAUSATION: THE 'BUT FOR' PRINCIPLE
Causation

There is another aspect that the patient must prove in order for their claim for compensation to succeed. There must be a causal link between the breach of duty of care and the harm suffered.

It is possible for a health professional to fail in their duty of care of a patient yet the health professional or employer might not be liable to the patient in civil law.

The patient (claimant) must prove that the defendant's breach of duty caused the harm. Two matters must be proved:

1 that as a fact, the defendant's breach caused the claimant's loss; and
2 the damage was not too remote.

The courts use the 'but for' test to determine whether the defendant caused the loss, that is, would the claimant have suffered loss but for the defendant's negligence? If the answer is 'no', then the defendant must logically have caused the harm and is liable.

This element of causation is often the most difficult legal hurdle for a patient to overcome when pursuing a claim for compensation.

EXAMPLE OF THE 'BUT FOR' PRINCIPLE

A patient is seen in the outpatient department and undergoes tests on a lump for suspected carcinoma. X-rays and other tests are undertaken.

Six months later the patient is re-referred by the GP and is again seen in the outpatient department. At this point they review the records and discover that the patient had been diagnosed with carcinoma six months previously, but for some reason the patient had fallen through the system. They now commence treatment.

Questions

➤ **Does the Trust owe the patient a duty of care?** Yes, the Trust owes the patient a duty of care.

➤ **Is the Trust in breach of the duty of care?** It is highly likely that the Trust will be in breach of the duty of care for failing to identify the diagnosis sooner and failing to treat the patient sooner. A responsible body of practitioners would say that they should not have failed to identify the diagnosis.

➤ **Did the breach of duty 'cause' the injury.** That is, did the failure to pick up on the diagnosis of carcinoma and delay in treatment cause the patient injury? The answer here is that the Trust did not cause the cancer. The patient already had cancer when he attended the hospital the first time.

➤ **So did the Trust 'cause' an injury because of the delay in treatment?** If the patient's condition when he was first seen six months before was that the cancer was slow growing and there was no risk of metastasising, what would the treatment have been? If, for example, the usual treatment in these circumstances would have been to commence treatment in six months' time, notwithstanding the delay, the treatment would have been the same as if they had made an immediate diagnosis and therefore the outcome would not have been any different.

In these circumstances, notwithstanding there was a delay in diagnosis and treatment, which constitutes a breach of duty of care, there is no causation and so any claim for compensation would fail.

If, however, the usual course of treatment would have been to commence treatment immediately but now, because of the delay in treatment, the cancer has metastasised, the patient needs further and more extensive surgery and life expectancy has been reduced, then the delay in treatment has caused the injury.

This is because 'but for' the delay in treatment the patient would not have gone on to suffer the cancer metastasising, would not have needed to undergo the further surgery and would not have a reduced life expectancy.

In these circumstances there is a causal link between the delay in diagnosis and the injury suffered. So causation would be proved for the purpose of a claim for compensation.

EXAMPLE OF CAUSATION

A female patient attends hospital complaining of severe stomach cramps. She is examined and tests are carried out. The doctor reassures the patient and says that she has probably eaten something that has upset her stomach and the patient is discharged. Two days later the patient is brought in by ambulance still complaining of severe stomach cramps. On review of the records it is clear that the patient is suffering from an ectopic pregnancy but the doctor had missed this on the previous occasion. The patient dies in the A&E before they can take her to theatre.

TASK

Questions
1 Is there a duty of care?
2 Did the defendant breach the duty of care? Would a responsible body of medical practitioners have acted in the same way?
3 Did the breach of duty of care cause the death of the patient? But for the actions of the doctor would the patient have survived?

Answers:
1 The Trust owes the patient a duty of care.
2 If the court were to determine that the responsible body of medical practitioners would have identified the ectopic pregnancy when the patient was first admitted then the doctor would be in breach of his duty of care. The court will then go on to consider causation: the 'but for' principle.
3 If the patient had been properly diagnosed and operated on the first day, would she have survived? If the court determines she would have survived if the doctor had properly diagnosed and treated her then the breach of duty caused the patient to die. The deceased's family would succeed in a claim for compensation.

A health professional owes a duty of care to the patient. If the standard of treatment falls short of what is expected then it may constitute a breach of duty of care. If, as a result, the patient is injured this may give rise to a claim for compensation.

You can see that the legal issues of causation are complex. If harm has occurred to a patient as a result of negligent care, they can seek compensation. However, not all harm will entitle the patient to compensation.

REASONABLY FORESEEABLE

In order to guard against risks, the outcome must be reasonably foreseeable. If the circumstances were not reasonable to foresee then negligence would not be established.

A nurse swabs the inside of a patient's mouth using cotton wool on the end of a pair of scissors! The very thought of this is cringeworthy! It is reasonably foreseeable that this practice could cause some harm.

CASE

Roe v Minister of Health 1954
A patient suffered severe injuries as a consequence of being given spinal anaesthetics. The anaesthetic agents were stored in glass ampoules and the ampoules themselves were kept in a solution of phenol. Unbeknown to anyone, the glass of the ampoules had invisible hairline cracks through which the

phenol penetrated, adulterating the anaesthetic agent and thus causing the injuries.

The patient sued, but lost the case. The possibility of seepage through invisible cracks was not known at the time. Therefore, it was not reasonably foreseeable that this might occur. However, if this should occur again the hospital would have difficulty in arguing that it was not reasonably foreseeable since the risks are now known.

Lord Denning in the case of Roe v Minister of Health 1954 stated:

> Medical science has conferred great benefits on mankind but these benefits are attended by considerable risks. Every surgical operation is attended by risks. We cannot take the benefits without taking the risks. Every advance in technique is also attended by risks. Doctors like the rest of us have to learn the hard way. Something goes wrong and shows up as a weakness, then it is put right . . . we must not look at a 1947 accident with 1954 spectacles.[9]

It follows that you can only guard against risks if they are known or reasonably likely to occur. If the reasonable person would not foresee a harmful consequence of an action, then a defendant will not be negligent in failing to take precautions.

The court will consider the likelihood of harm occurring. The greater the risk of harm the greater the precautions that will need to be taken.

Too remote

It must be established that the harm caused as a result of negligence must not be too remote.

EXAMPLES OF 'TOO REMOTE'

Example 1

If a person is in a car and someone crashes into them and causes them an injury, for example a whiplash, then there is a claim.

But if, whilst a person is on a motorway, there is an accident and they are not hit but are stuck in the traffic jam caused by the accident, they may lose half a day's pay as a result. But there is no claim. This is because the act is too remote, it is not close enough.

Example 2

A gentleman was injured in a road traffic accident. Negligence was admitted. As part of his claim he recovered money for care and he went to the south coast to receive the care he needed. Whilst he was at the south coast he fell over and suffered a fracture. He said had he not had the original accident he would not have been at the south coast recuperating and thus he would not have suffered an injury.

He lost the claim for this from the car driver who caused the road traffic accident as it was not directly connected; it was too remote.

Thin skull rule

There is an exception to the rule of reasonable foreseeability, which is the 'thin skull rule'. In other words, you take your victim as you find them.

EXAMPLE OF 'THIN SKULL RULE'

The patient has an unusually thin skull. The patient falls off the MRI scanner bed and bumps his head. It is a minor bump but the patient suffers a serious fracture because of his thin skull and dies as a result.

The health professional is in breach of the duty of care, and is therefore negligent in allowing the patient to fall from the MRI bed. You cannot claim that although you were negligent in the patient falling from the scanner bed, you did not cause the death because usually such a minor injury would not result in death and that the death was caused because the patient had a thin skull.

In this scenario the health professional is negligent. Even though the outcome could not have been anticipated the health professional would be liable for the harm caused because of the application of the 'thin skull rule': you must take your victim as you find them.

This principle applies to all situations – not just those involving a skull.

DEFENCES TO CLAIMS FOR NEGLIGENCE
No defence

EXAMPLE OF NO DEFENCE

A mother was in a hospital waiting room when her small child went behind her chair and put his hand on a hot water pipe. The mother rushed him to the toilet, which happened to be a staff toilet, and ran his hand under the cold tap. The tap was wrongly marked 'cold' and very hot water came of the tap and over the child's hand causing serious burns. The hospital said it was a staff toilet and not for use by patients and that the staff knew the tap was wrongly marked.

The court said there was no defence.

Res ipsa loquitur – the thing speaks for itself

There are occasions where the circumstances are so obvious that the thing speaks for itself.

For example, if a wheel falls off an ambulance then it speaks for itself that it is the fault of the ambulance Trust; the vehicle should have been properly maintained.

Consent

If a person is advised of the risks of a procedure and voluntarily accepts the risk, but during surgery a known risk manifests, they cannot then make a claim.

Consent becomes important. Consent can be by implication, written or verbal.

It is preferable though to make a written record. Consent is a complex area and the health professional should be fully conversant with it.

Contributory negligence

Where a patient contributes to the harm caused the judge may reduce an award to reflect this. This is expressed as a percentage contribution.

EXAMPLE OF CONTRIBUTORY NEGLIGENCE

A patient is brought into the A&E Department having tripped and hurt their ankle. They are x-rayed and advised that it is a sprain and they should rest it and not to bear weight on it.

A week later the patient returns still in pain. The x-ray is reviewed and a fracture is noted, which had been overlooked previously. The patient's ankle required a plaster cast. However, because of the delay in diagnosing and the fact that the patient has been weight bearing, the fracture has worsened. It now requires a longer course of treatment than it would have done had it been properly diagnosed and treated on admission a week earlier.

In these circumstances the court would consider that the hospital was negligent in not diagnosing and treating the fracture sooner. However, they would also consider that the patient contributed to the damage caused because he was weight bearing when he had been advised not to. The patient would have contributed to his injury. The court might apportion 50% contributory negligence to the patient.

In these circumstances any compensation claimed would be reduced by 50% to reflect the patient contributing to his own injury.

CALCULATING COMPENSATION/DAMAGES

A patient who suffers harm as a result of negligent clinical treatment may be entitled to be compensated for any financial loss they suffered as a consequence. This is referred to as 'compensation' or 'damages'.

The purpose of the claim is for the injured party to be compensated. Its purpose is not to punish the negligent person or organisation. It is to place the injured party in the financial position he would have been in had the injury or damage not occurred. If there is no loss then there is no claim.

Compensation is made of two parts. 'General damages' for the pain and suffering and 'special damages' for expenses.

General damages

General damages in England and Wales are not very high compared to the USA or Ireland, for example. They are calculated using case law and the Judicial Studies Board Guideline (JSB)[10] as a rule of thumb. The JSB sets out a range of compensation, such as for the loss of a leg, loss of an eye, scarring and so on.

Special damages

Special damages are the expenses and financial loss incurred. These include items such as loss of earnings, the need for nursing care, help around the home and garden, medication, equipment and adaptations to the home.

It is the special damages that are often the highest part of the claim and in some cases this can run into millions of pounds. In birth trauma cases the special damages are usually very high due to the level of medical and nursing support the child will need for the rest of their life. Each case can cost the Trusts on average between £3 million and £5.5 million.

EXAMPLE OF SPECIAL DAMAGES

A female patient 30 years of age attends hospital for investigation for a breast lump. She is diagnosed as having grade I carcinoma. She receives three courses of chemotherapy treatment. The hospital subsequently discovers it had the wrong results for the patient and that she had a lipoma, which did not require any treatment.

The hospital's negligence caused the patient injury and loss and the patient is entitled to compensation.

Value of the claim

HOW MUCH IS THE PATIENT ENTITLED TO?

The patient did not have cancer but a lipoma. If she had been treated appropriately she would have been told about her condition and would not have required any treatment. There would have been no impact on her work or family life.

As she received chemotherapy treatment she was unable to work. She suffered side effects of chemotherapy including hair loss, sickness, fatigue, permanent damage to her immune system and she is now infertile. She required hospital admission during the treatment, which made her very unwell. She was unable to return to work. Damage to her immune system has left her very weak and she requires help around the home and adaptations to the home. She is devastated that she is now unable to have any children. She is unable to return to work.

'General damages' is for pain and suffering. In this scenario it would be for the pain and suffering, hair loss, damage to immune system and the fact that she cannot have any children.

'Special damages' would include loss of earnings, rehabilitation, help around the home to assist with cooking, cleaning and gardening, adaptations to the home, such as hand rails in the bathroom and a chair lift.

Claims may arise out of the same type of negligence but the compensation for each may vary hugely. For example, in the cases of patients whose legs have been amputated by mistake, one patient's claim may be worth only £10 000 including both general and special damages. If that patient was immobile prior to the amputation, was not working and never likely to work, then there has been little financial impact as a result of the negligence; whereas another patient's claim might be millions of pounds if they are a professional footballer at the peak of their career whose loss of income would be significant.

If a patient dies

If a patient dies as a result of negligence the claimant may be entitled to a 'bereavement award' currently fixed by law at £10 000.[11] In addition, they may be entitled to the funeral costs and loss of dependency.

A claim may be made by the personal representative in the estate, or the relatives and/or dependants of the deceased.

The definition of a dependant is set down in statute.[12] It is someone who was reliant upon the deceased's income and must be one of the following:

➤ the spouse or former spouse
➤ co-habitants, providing they meet certain criteria
➤ the parents or other ascendants of the deceased
➤ any person whom the deceased treated as a parent
➤ the children or other descendants of the deceased
➤ any person whom not being the deceased's own child by reason of marriage was treated by the deceased as a child of the family
➤ the brother, sister, uncle or aunt of the deceased.

A dependency claim would apply where, for example, there was a reliance on the deceased's earnings or they were providing care.

Review task

REVIEW OF THE SCENARIO

Tom, a keen gardener, also makes homebrew in his garden shed. Having enjoyed a glass of his homebrew he invites his next-door neighbor, Bill, into his garden shed for a tipple of his homebrew.

Bill has a better idea, 'Why don't we go to the pub instead?' Off they go to the pub and they order half a pint of beer each. Tom takes a sip of his beer and says 'I don't feel very well.' Bill says 'You look terrible I think you ought to go to the hospital.'

They arrive at the accident and emergency department and Tom is triaged by the nurse. Tom tells the nurse 'I had a tipple of my homebrew and then we went to the pub.' The nurse tells Tom 'You are drunk, go home and sleep it off. If you are not better by the morning go and see your GP.'

By the morning Tom was dead. Tom had inadvertently drunk paraquat in his garden shed. An assumption had been made by the triage nurse that Tom was drunk.

Do you think Tom's family would succeed in claiming compensation?

Questions

➤ **Was there a duty of care?** Yes a duty of care was owed to Tom.

➤ **Did the triage nurse breach the duty of care? Would a responsible body of medical practitioners have acted in the same way? That is, would a responsible body of triage nurses have acted in the same way?** The nurse should have taken a proper history and not made an assumption that the patient was drunk. Proper tests should have been carried out to determine or rule out any other cause. Blood test results would have revealed poison and the nurse should have taken advice from the poisons unit. No responsible body of medical practitioners would have acted in the way the nurse did and therefore the nurse is in breach of the duty of care.

➤ **Did the breach of duty of care cause the death of the patient? 'But for' the actions of the triage nurse would the patient have survived?** The patient died of paraquat poisoning. There is no known antidote for this. Even if the nurse had carried out the correct procedure there was little they could have done for this patient; the patient would have died in any event. There is no causal link between the negligence and the cause of death.

➤ **Was it reasonably foreseeable?** It is reasonably foreseeable that if an assumption is made that the patient was drunk without proper investigations then something might be missed, which could cause the patient harm.

➤ **Was there loss?** The patient died so there was loss. The deceased estate would be entitled to bring a claim.

From this scenario you may be surprised to read that this claim would not succeed. This is because there was no 'causation'. All of the legal elements must be established for the claim to succeed.

Recap

In order for a patient to succeed in a claim for compensation they have to establish:

1 that the defendant owed them a duty of care
2 that the defendant breached that duty of care
3 that such breach caused the injury or loss, known as 'causation'
4 that the injury was 'reasonably foreseeable'
5 and that as a result the claimant has suffered loss.

Remember, an adverse outcome alone is not in itself sufficient for a patient who has been injured to succeed in claiming compensation. All of the legal elements need to be present for any such claim to succeed.

Where there is an adverse outcome the health professional will be accountable in all areas. Whilst a claim for compensation may not succeed, the health professional will still be accountable to his professional body, employer and society. For example criminal charges may still be brought; they may be brought before their professional body who may strike them from the register and/or the employer may discipline or dismiss them.

REFERENCES

1 Civil Procedure Rules 1998.
2 Limitation Act 1980.
3 Donoghue v Stevenson (1932) All ER Rep 1; 1932 AC 562.
4 R v South West London and St George's Mental Health Trust 2007 EWCA Civ 106, CA.

5   Kent v Griffiths and Others 1998, (2001) QB 36, (2000) 2 All ER 474; (2000) 2 WLR 1158, (2000) Lloyd's Rep Med 109; (2000) 07 LS Gaz R 41; (2000) NLJR 195; 144 Sol Jo LB 106.
6   Phelps v Hillingdon London Borough Council (1998) 1 All ER 421.
7   Bolam v Friern Barnet 1957 2 All ER 118.
8   Whitehouse v Jordan 1981 1 All ER 267.
9   Roe v Minister of Health 1954 2 AER 131.
10 Judicial Studies Board. *Guidelines for the Assessment of General Damages in Personal Injury.* London: Judicial Studies Board; 2006.
11 Fatal Accidents Act 1976, as amended by the Administration of Justice Act 1982.
12 Law Reform (Miscellaneous Provisions) Act 1934, as amended by the Administration of Justice Act 1982.

CHAPTER 9

When a patient complains

There are an increasing number of complaints made against the NHS each year. For some this is a bad sign and indicative of a growing discontent with the health service; whereas to others it is an opportunity to improve the service.

It is highly likely that a health professional sometime during their career will be involved in a complaint, either in relation to their own work or a complaint about someone else's.

Complaints may arise, for example, out of a poor bedside manner, rudeness or lack of information. The main cause of clinical accidents is a breakdown in communication, mainly through poor documentation, poor records, system failures and consent issues. When a clinical accident happens, a very high proportion of patients will pursue a claim because of a poor handling of the complaints procedure. Patients sometimes feel that there was a failure to address the issues; that there was a cover up; that they are hiding something; that they are sweeping it under the carpet. There is often a fear on the part of the Trust of saying 'I'm sorry'. If the patient's issues have not been addressed, their only recourse to find the answers is through the legal process. This then becomes time consuming and costly and causes additional anxiety to the patient and the health professionals involved.

Of course it is far better to avoid complaints by improving record keeping, addressing system failures and so on, but when something has gone wrong, dealing with the complaint effectively is paramount.

All complaints, whether oral or written, should receive a positive and full response, with the aim of satisfying the complainant that his/her concerns have been heeded, and offering an apology and explanation as appropriate, and referring to any remedial action that will follow.

The Trust's chief executive will be responsible for ensuring that there is appropriate local policy and procedural guidance in place that is available to all staff.

Where a patient is dissatisfied about their care or treatment or if they have suffered an injury as a result of treatment they received, the patient has several options in pursuing their complaint. These options include an informal or formal complaint to the Trust or organisation responsible, reporting the matter to the professional body, seeking legal advice from a solicitor and suing the Trust, or pursuing compensation through the 'redress scheme'.[1]

Health authorities are required to have in place a complaints procedure. Local Authority Social Services and National Health Service Complaints (England) Regulations 2009 came into force on 1 April 2009.[2]

INFORMAL COMPLAINT

An informal complaint may best be described as 'a concern'. A patient might raise a concern with a health professional when passing in a corridor or at the bedside or they may have specifically asked to speak to someone to discuss their concerns.

Informal complaints usually involve matters such as lack of information. But when does a 'concern' become a complaint?

An informal complaint or concern can be distinguished from a formal complaint by the nature of the complaint. If the complaint requires some intervention then it is likely to be formal.

EXAMPLE OF AN INFORMAL COMPLAINT

Following surgery, a patient is told that he is ready for discharge and the staff explain that there are signs and symptoms to look out for and that they will give him a leaflet explaining this before he goes home.

They fail to give him the leaflet and the patient asks the staff on two occasions for the leaflet but they still don't give it to him. The patient complains.

This is an informal complaint (i.e. a concern) and can quite easily be dealt with by giving the patient the leaflet and apologising.

If the matter is not dealt with it could turn into a formal complaint.

FORMAL COMPLAINT

EXAMPLE OF A FORMAL COMPLAINT

In similar circumstances, following surgery, a patient is told that he is ready for discharge and the staff explain that there are signs and symptoms to look out for and that they will give him a leaflet explaining this before he goes home.

They fail to give him the leaflet and the patient asks the staff on two occasions for the leaflet, but they still don't give it to him.

The patient is discharged home and he develops a headache, dizziness and nausea for a period of four days. He considers this not to be very significant. Having just had surgery he thinks this is probably to be expected. He collapses at home and an ambulance takes him back to the hospital. He is suffering from adverse side effects of medication.

The hospital inform him that he should have contacted them immediately as his symptoms were signs that something was wrong and that he should have been told what to look out for. The patient sends a letter of complaint.

This is more likely to be considered as a formal complaint. This requires intervention. An internal investigation to see why the patient was not given the information he required should be undertaken. A formal written response should be given to the patient.

A formal complaint does not necessarily have to be put in writing by a patient.

If, having pursued the formal complaint process, the patient is not satisfied with the response, the patient may appeal to the ombudsman.

PROFESSIONAL BODY

A patient might not necessarily inform the care provider of their complaint. They may go directly to the professional body. The professional body will then take up the matter and they will correspond directly with the patient. They will investigate the complaint and take all necessary steps, which will be to call into account those health professionals involved in the patient's care. This process calls into account the health professional's ability but the patient cannot use this process to claim financial compensation.

LEGAL ADVICE/CLAIM

The patient may go directly to a solicitor for advice on whether the care they received was negligent. The patient may have already been through the complaint process with the care provider, but may not be satisfied with the response.

The solicitor will advise the patient on whether there is a potential claim for negligence and whether they may be entitled to compensation. This process is dealt with in detail in Chapter 8.

THE NHS REDRESS ACT 2007

The NHS Redress Act 2007[3] received royal assent in November 2006. The act sets out a framework for redress, the guidelines of which are yet to be finalised. The scheme has not yet been implemented and there is no precise time frame for commencement of the scheme, but it is anticipated that it will be April 2009.

The aim of the scheme is to provide a more speedy resolution to a claim with more consistent outcomes and to set up a framework to provide an investigation, apology, compensation, and care (where appropriate) without the need to go through the court process. It is hoped that the scheme will establish a more open and fair culture in the NHS and that it will ensure that lessons are learned from mistakes.

This scheme will deal with claims that are valued at less than £20 000. Once the patient has opted to go through the redress scheme they cannot then change their minds later and go through the court process. They must choose which avenue to take at the outset. If they do not succeed in obtaining compensation through the redress scheme the court process will not become open to them later.

REFERENCES

1 NHS Redress Act 2007.
2 Local Authority Social Services and National Health Service Complaints (England) Regulations 2009, SI 2009 no 309. Available at: www.opsi.gov.uk/si/si2009/uksi_20090309_en_1 (accessed 27 April 2009).
3 NHS Redress Act, op. cit.

CHAPTER 10

Human rights

The European Convention on Human Rights (ECHR) was incorporated into English law with the Human Rights Act 1998.[1] The Act did not open the floodgates to a myriad of claims as had been anticipated and so there is very little case law on the subject as it relates to health or anything else. Although the Act is divided into sections, it is customary to refer to the Articles of the ECHR when discussing it.

In brief the Human Rights Act gives individuals rights within society. There is a duty on government to enforce and protect those rights. The ECHR states that an organisation of the state (like the NHS) owes patients and clients a responsibility to maintain and uphold human rights.

Health professionals also have a duty to uphold patients' human rights, but if they fail to do so they will be accountable to their professional body and could face disciplinary action by the employer.

Private hospitals are not organisations of the state, so technically they are not bound by the Act. However, they are providing a public service and will therefore be caught by the Act. Health professionals working in the private health sector will be expected to have regard to the Act under their contractual obligations.

The Human Rights Act is not designed to facilitate access to healthcare or medical information. Its purpose is to protect the individual against state action. However, health professionals must always have regard to the Human Rights Act when treating and caring for patients.

Health professionals should presume that almost all decisions about healthcare will have some potential impact upon somebody's human rights and as a result it is imperative to ensure that the reasoning for reaching any adverse decision is clear.

The Articles of the ECHR that health professionals will be mainly concerned with are:

➤ **Article 2** – 'Everyone's right to life shall be protected by law'
➤ **Article 3** – 'No one shall be subjected to torture or to inhuman or degrading treatment or punishment'
➤ **Article 8** – 'Everyone has the right to respect for his private and family life, his home and his correspondence.'

ARTICLE 2: 'EVERYONE'S RIGHT TO LIFE SHALL BE PROTECTED BY LAW'

This imposes a duty not only to refrain from interfering with life, but also a 'positive duty to take appropriate steps to safeguard life'.[2]

It has been suggested that this could be used where resources are refused or treatment is withdrawn or withheld, such as a decision not to resuscitate.

CASE

National Health Service Trust A v D and others (2000)
Parents of a severely disabled baby challenged a 'not for resuscitation' (NFR) decision. The court, however, held that full palliative care recommended by the doctors, such as pain relief, allowing the baby to die with dignity, was not a breach of Article 2.[3]

ARTICLE 3: 'NO ONE SHALL BE SUBJECTED TO TORTURE OR TO INHUMAN OR DEGRADING TREATMENT OR PUNISHMENT'

It has been argued that this right might be infringed where a patient is left on a stretcher in the corridor for several hours or in issues of manual handling where hoists are being used.[4]

However, such cases are unlikely to succeed. Article 3 imposes a high threshold; the conditions to which the individual risks being exposed must be severe for him to get home under this Article.

CASE

D v United Kingdom (1997)
A convicted drug trafficker in the terminal stages of AIDS was threatened with deportation to the Island of St Kitts. The court accepted the argument that the absence of vital medical treatment would rapidly accelerate his death and that this breached Article 3.[5]

ARTICLE 8: 'EVERYONE HAS THE RIGHT TO RESPECT FOR HIS PRIVATE AND FAMILY LIFE, HIS HOME AND HIS CORRESPONDENCE'

For health professionals this concerns the issues of confidentiality of medical information. Any public authority which collects, holds, processes and withholds from an individual certain personal information such as medical data will be interfering with their private life.

Article 8 relates not only to the right of an individual to prevent others from seeing medical information about him, but also to his right to see that information for himself. In most cases, access is provided for by statute like, for example, the Access to Health Records Act 1990[6] and the Data Protection Act 1998,[7] with statutory exemptions in the case where release of the information to the patient would be likely to cause serious physical or psychological harm to that patient.

CONSENT AND HUMAN RIGHTS

The issue of consent is reliant upon access to information because consent depends on the quality of the information given to the patient.

CASE

Sidaway
In this case the House of Lords decided that a doctor's duty to inform the patient is an aspect of the doctor's duty to exercise reasonable care and skill, and not an aspect of the patient's right to know.

The content of the duty is governed wholly by the Bolam principle according to which a doctor must pass on to the patient that information which is thought appropriate by a responsible body of medical opinion.[8]

There is a clear difference between information which, if withheld from the patient, would not result in negligence and information to which the patient is reasonably entitled in order to make an informed decision. The test is what the reasonably competent doctor regards as being significant on the one hand and what the reasonably ordinary patient regards as being of importance on the other.

PATIENTS' RIGHT TO PRIVACY

Other issues may arise under Article 8, such as the presence of several student doctors at the examination of a patient, or leaving patients on trolleys in corridors or other areas in which they may be viewed by members of the public.[9,10]

REFERENCES

1 Human Rights Act 1998.
2 Association X v UK Application No 7154/75 (1978) 14 DR 31.
3 National Health Service Trust A v D and others 2000 Lloyd's Rep Med 411 706.
4 R v (1) East Sussex County Council (2) The Disability Rights Commission (Interested Party), exparte A, B 2003 EWHC 167 (Admin); (2003) 6 CCLR 194, at paras [178]–[185].
5 D v United Kingdom 1997 24 EHRR 423.
6 Access to Health Records Act 1990.
7 Data Protection Act 1998.
8 Sidaway v Bethlem Royal Hospital Governors and others 1985 1All ER 643.
9 A v B PLC and Another 2002 3 WLR 542.
10 R v Secretary of State for The Home Department, Ex parte Daley 2001 1WLR 2099.

CHAPTER 11

Risk management

*'We were short staffed, I was under
pressure, but I meant well.'*

In the course of everyday practice, health professionals are making decisions about the care, planning and treatment of a patient. When doing so they are balancing the risks. We are often faced with difficult dilemmas particularly as there is a reliance on a network of others, and matters that the health professional has no control over, such as lack of resources.

Good risk management is asking 'what if' and putting procedures in place to avoid accidents and errors. It is not good risk management if measures are implemented as a result of an audit or an incident.

Of course when something goes wrong it must be addressed. As a lawyer it is very frustrating to see the same incidents occurring time and again. Clinical accidents cause devastation to the patients, their families and also for the health professionals involved. The cost of clinical errors is huge, running into billions of pounds. Imagine the resources that could be purchased with that sort of money instead.

Health professionals are concerned with what happens to them when something goes wrong and who will be responsible. In particular, they are concerned with matters involving delegation, team decisions, following orders, protocols and guidelines, lack of training, lack of supervision, or supervising others, an emergency, working long hours, and covering several wards. Who is responsible in these circumstances?

It is important to remember that the law applies strictly. Be under no illusion, the judge will have no sympathy for a health professional who causes injury to a patient because they were tired, understaffed, did not have adequate resources, were not trained appropriately or were told to do a particular thing.

Another important aspect is that health professionals should be familiar with the law that applies to them in their area such as the Mental Health Act 1983,[1] which all mental health practitioners should be aware of. It is the responsibility of health professionals to keep abreast of changes in the law that impact on their own practice. Remember, ignorance of the law is no defence.

CLINICAL GOVERNANCE

Clinical governance is a framework designed to help healthcare professionals to continuously improve quality and safeguard standards of care.

The principles of clinical governance, launched in 1998 within the NHS, apply equally within the independent and private sectors, as supported by the Care Standards Act 2000.[2]

Clinical governance helps to maintain and improve the high standards of professional practice expected from health professionals. This is achieved through quality assurance initiatives such as:

➤ clinical audit
➤ evidence-based practice
➤ clinical supervision
➤ research
➤ complaints and critical incident reporting.

Such initiatives highlight good practice and identify where improvements are required.

Clinical governance is underpinned by:

➤ professional self-regulation
➤ strong leadership
➤ effective communication
➤ being patient focused
➤ commitment to quality
➤ valuing each other
➤ continuing professional development.

The application of these principles provides an environment in which clinical excellence can flourish and high standards of patient care can be promoted. Clinical governance provides the framework to assist in the co-ordination of these activities to produce quality initiatives focused on improving patient care.[3]

AUTHORITY, SKILL, ABILITY AND COMPETENCE

Health professionals' practice must be sensitive, relevant and responsive to the needs of individual patients and have the capacity to adjust, where and when appropriate, to changing circumstances.

Health professionals must maintain their professional knowledge and competence. This includes undertaking regular activities to develop competence and performance. Health professionals must be aware of their limitations and ensure that they are competent to undertake their activities. If they are not then they must obtain help and supervision until they are considered by both themselves and the employer to be competent to carry out the task.

Certain codes of conduct provide that the health professional must undertake a certain number of refresher days. Health professionals must be aware of any such requirement either by their professional body, employer or under any other rules that apply to them.

The employer must be confident that the health professional is capable of carrying out their activities. The employer must be satisfied that the health professional has the authority, skill, ability and competence to carry out such tasks.

Authority

Do you have authority from your employer to carry out the task?

This will be determined by the contract of employment and job description. Those documents set out the roles and responsibilities. If a health professional carries out duties that are not contained within the contract of employment and job description then they could be in breach of contract.

Health professionals should look carefully at their job description. Check if it provides for job development. Your job description should be reviewed in the light of changes in authority. Quite often the last clause in a job description states along the lines of '. . . and anything you are required to do'. It should be clear and unambiguous so that you are not faced with a problem after an event when the employer says, 'that's not what it means'.

Authority is a matter for the employer. They will set down what you can and cannot do.

Skill and ability

Do you have the skill and ability to carry out the task?

Your skill and ability is demonstrated by your qualifications and experience. If you hold yourself out as having the skill and ability, it is the employer's responsibility to validate that you do. You will inform them of your skill and ability and they will check your qualifications and certificates.

They will be aware of ongoing training and supervision. The employer may arrange for further training and education or you may have arranged it yourself. You will inform the employer of your ongoing education and training and a file should be held of all such activities.

Demonstrating skill and ability is the joint responsibility of the health professional and the employer.

Competence

Do you have the competence to carry out the task?

Competence can be defined as: 'the state of having the knowledge, judgement, skills, energy, experience and motivation required to respond adequately to the demands of one's professional responsibilities'.

A health professional may have the authority to carry out certain tasks; they may have the skill and ability, but do they have the competence?

The health professional must know the limits of their competency and only undertake tasks and accept responsibilities for those tasks for which they are competent. Even though they may have had the training it may be many months or indeed years since they practised in the area; for example, they may have been out of practice through maternity leave or a sabbatical.

Many things can impact on competency. Notwithstanding you have the certificate it may be that you have only carried out the procedure once and you would need to be supervised before you can do it alone. It may be that whilst usually you would be competent you are feeling unwell and that the procedure requires a great deal of concentration, which you do not have that day. It is for you to know if you have the competency. The employer will not be aware of this unless you tell them. There is no point after an incident has occurred to say, 'well I wasn't feeling well'. In order to risk manage, the employer needs to know so they may make other provisions for the patient.

If a task is beyond your level of competence or outside your professional area you must obtain help and supervision from a competent practitioner until you and the employer are satisfied that you are competent.

It is a little like driving a car. You have authority to drive if you hold a driving licence. Skill and ability is evidenced by passing your driving test. Competence is a matter for you. If you are tired or have consumed alcohol, this will adversely affect the way you drive. Driving a manual car when you are used to an automatic can be a problem. You must recognise your limitations.

Employers have a responsibility to ensure they have systems in place to facilitate the early detection of a lack of competence. Such systems must include further training and support as necessary within a given time frame in order to help the health professional achieve the required competency. Where the lack of competency cannot be managed, staff should be aware of the reporting process to the professional bodies.

Authority, skill, ability and competence – if these are missing you will not be discharging your duty of care. This will give rise to both legal and professional sanctions.

REFUSING TO UNDERTAKE A TASK

We have seen previously how a health professional must have the authority, skill and ability to carry out the task in hand. They must know the limits of their competency.

A health professional might have to refuse to undertake a task where he is not properly trained to perform it or, for example, where he has insufficient time to carry it out safely.

BALANCING THE RISKS

In the everyday role of the health professional we are weighing up and balancing the risks when making decisions about patient care, planning, treatment and support. This is not always easy. Treatment confers great benefits but these benefits are often attended by considerable risks. We cannot always bestow the benefits without taking the risks. With hindsight we might have done things differently as it is easy to be wise after the event.

The health professional must consider the risks and weigh them up. The health professional must justify their actions. The process, the decision and the rationale for doing so must be recorded in the health records.

TASK

Consider the use of cot sides when caring for elderly patients.

■ One nurse will say 'I always use them'
■ Another will say 'I never use them'.

Who is right?

They are both wrong; they are not making a risk assessment.

The nurse who always uses cot sides will be negligent if they are not suitable for a patient because, for example, the patient is known to thrash around and could therefore harm themselves on the cot sides.

The nurse who never uses cot sides would be equally negligent if the patient fell out of bed three nights in a row and the nurse did not review it and did nothing about it.

A decision carries with it both risks and benefits. You must make the decision based upon your knowledge of the patient.

EXAMPLE OF DEGREE OF RISK

A patient is admitted into hospital with a provisional diagnosis of meningitis. The patient is immediately barrier nursed in a single room, even though that means moving a very sick patient to a four-bed ward. The patient who was moved died in the night. The family of the deceased criticised the hospital for moving the patient and suggested that the move accelerated the patient's death.

TASK

Was the nurse at fault for moving the patient to the four-bed ward?

Was the nurse at fault if the patient with suspected meningitis was found to be suffering only from a non-fatal virus?

Provided the nurse used her professional judgement in making the decision to give the single room to the particular patient, with the knowledge available to her at the time, then there should be no finding of negligence.

In fact, if the patient had been diagnosed with meningitis, the nurse may well have been negligent in not taking precautions to prevent danger of staff and patients becoming infected.

The nurse has to use his judgement in determining the degree of risk to both patients.

A health professional must balance the risks and can do so based only on the information available to them at the time. However, it is not an excuse to say 'I didn't have the records or the x-ray.' That information is available and if something goes wrong because the health professional failed to read the records or obtain them, they will be responsible.

REFUSING TO UNDERTAKE TRAINING

The roles of many health professionals have become much wider. The role of ambulance staff has been extended into 'emergency care practitioners'. The role of prescribing for non-medical practitioners, such as pharmacists and other allied health professionals, and the role of nurses have expanded.

It is usually required that health professionals must keep their knowledge and skills up-to-date throughout their working life. It could therefore be said that it would be inappropriate for health professionals to refuse to develop their professional practice beyond the level they reached on qualifying.

If the employer wishes the health professional to take on new tasks then it is a contractual requirement of the employer to ensure that health professionals are competent to perform the tasks they are asked to undertake. The employer must therefore ensure that adequate training is provided and undertaken.

CONTINUING EDUCATION AND KEEPING UP-TO-DATE

It is a requirement that health professionals keep their knowledge and skills up-to-date throughout their working life. How far and how often are they expected to update their knowledge?

CASE

Crawford v Charing Cross Hospital

In the case of Crawford v Charing Cross Hospital, a patient developed brachial palsy in an arm following a blood transfusion. The patient brought a claim and at first the court said the hospital was negligent on the basis of an article published in *The Lancet* six months previously, setting out this hazard.

However, the hospital appealed and the Court of Appeal overturned this decision, saying it would be too great a burden to expect a doctor to read every article in medical journals.[4]

The courts may be reluctant to convict on the basis of one article, but where a particular risk has been highlighted on a number of occasions, it will be difficult to defend an action where a practitioner has not taken this into account.

However, articles in journals can have differing status. Some are just for research and have not yet been embraced into acceptable practice. Others are controversial and may never be adopted as recognised practice. Some may have direct and immediate effect, such as a directive from the Department of Health or, for example, from the Committee for Safety of Medicines, warning against prescribing a particular drug. To ignore these is likely to be deemed negligent.

NEW AND DEVELOPING PRACTICES

It may be comfortable for a health professional to hold onto old practices that they are familiar with. However, a health professional cannot hold onto old practices where medicine has moved on.

In the case of Bolam v Friern Hospital, the judge stated that a doctor cannot:

> . . . obstinately and pig-headedly carry on with some old technique if it has been proved to be contrary to what is really substantially the whole of informed medical opinion.[5]

Where practice has moved on then you cannot hold onto old practice. You must embrace the new practice.

Conversely, it is inappropriate for a health professional to go off on a frolic of their own and consider something they have read in a journal, for example, they might think 'this sounds like a good idea' and decide to implement it. Some practices may not have been embraced into acceptable practice and some may never become recognised practice.

EXAMPLE OF A HEALTH PROFESSIONAL FROLIC

A senior community midwife performed circumcisions on newborn babies, at the request of parents. She said, 'One day all midwives will be doing this; I am ahead of my time.'

The midwife kept good notes. However, nothing in the notes referred to the fact she had been carrying out the circumcisions.

The midwife must follow acceptable standards of practice. The midwife was reported to the professional body. She failed to record the treatment she had in fact carried out. It follows that she knew she should not have done it.

If it had been recorded the question would be: why didn't the supervisor pick it up?

Difficulties arise when health professionals are working on the cutting edge of practice. Where there are new developments you need to have professional support behind you. There should be peer review and it should be endorsed by the profession.

INEXPERIENCE

The same standard of care is expected of a junior or newly qualified health professional as that of an experienced one, but in practice it is impossible to expect the same standard of care. However, the courts do not make an allowance for 'trainees' when assessing liability.

CASE

Nettleship v Western

This case concerned a learner driver. The court determined that people who are learning a skill must exercise the same standard of care as those who are already proficient in that skill. A trainee's 'incompetent best' is not good enough.[6]

This may seem harsh but it is essential for public confidence. Legally the patient is entitled to the same level of acceptable care regardless of whether the health professional is a junior or senior. It is no defence to say the reason that the patient was given the wrong treatment was because the health professional was newly qualified.

CASE

Jones v Manchester Corporation

In this case the Court of Appeal held that inexperience was no defence when a patient died from an excessive dose of anaesthetic administered by an inexperienced doctor.[7]

In order to ensure that safe practice is undertaken, it is imperative that health professionals are competent, and that care which requires a greater degree of experience must be carried out by those appropriately skilled and competent. Those health professionals lacking in skills need to be adequately supervised.

APPROVED PRACTICES

Whether the care provided by a health professional is negligent or not will be judged on the reasonable standard of care, as set out in the Bolam principle discussed in Chapter 8.

The test as to whether health professionals are in breach of their duty of care is whether a responsible body of medical practitioners would have acted in the same way. Thus the negligence of a health professional, such as a nurse, will be determined by the standard of the ordinary skilled nurse. They will look at what is the approved practice of a nurse.

Outside the context of clinical negligence the courts have had no difficulty with the concept that commonly adopted practices may be negligent.

CASE

Edward Wong Finance Company Ltd v Johnson Stokes and Masters
This approach is demonstrated in Edward Wong Finance Company Ltd v Johnson Stokes and Masters where the Privy Council held that a particular conveyancing practice widely followed in Hong Kong was negligent despite the fact that virtually all other solicitors adopted the same practice.[8]

CASE

The Herald of Free Enterprise
Similarly, in this case the Divisional Court of Appeal stated that the practice of failing to check that the doors had been closed was prevalent in most if not all ferries of that class.

The Court concluded, however, that this was not evidence of the appropriate standard of care, but a failure to apply common sense in respect of elementary precautions required for the safety of the ship and that the common practice was negligent.[9]

The appropriate standard of care and whether a health professional has met that standard are crucial issues in determining a negligence action. The court has to decide if the health professional has exercised sufficient care. The test for breach of duty of care is whether or not the health professional's conduct was reasonable taking all the circumstances into account. Expert medical opinion is obviously important in assisting the courts to decide whether or not the health professional has exercised an appropriate level of skill in the circumstances of the case, but it is the courts and not expert medical opinion that decide if the health professional has achieved that standard.[10]

The effect of this is that notwithstanding the health professional may follow the practice adopted by others, the court may nevertheless deem that practice to be negligent.

EXAMPLE OF COLLECTIVE NEGLIGENT PRACTICE

A midwife administers an epidural to a patient. It causes paralysis. The midwife does not hold a certificate of competency in the administration of epidurals. She says there is only one midwife who has a certificate and it is not practical for her to carry out all of the epidurals herself. She would not have the time and anyway she is not always on duty. She says that nearly all the midwives she works with carry out the epidural even though they do not have certificates of competency. She says that it is acceptable practice on her ward – they all do it.

The fact that all the midwives carry out the procedure without certificates does not make it an approved practice from the court's point of view and the midwife can be held to be negligent.

DEVIATION FROM APPROVED PRACTICES

Approved practices have developed with the minimising of risks in mind. Such practices should be followed. Professional bodies, employers and patients expect that approved practices will be followed. If they are not, the health professional will be called to account.

However, where a health professional departs from approved practices it does not necessarily follow that this is evidence of negligence. There may be very good reasons why an approved practice has not been followed. Where the health professionals depart from approved practice they must be able to justify their actions. Deviation from approved practice should be well documented with all the facts and reasons why included.

CASE

Maynard v West Midlands Regional Health Authority 1985
In this case, two consultants thought that a female patient with a chest complaint might have tuberculosis, but they also considered the possibility of Hodgkin's disease. Before obtaining the result of a test, which would have

determined whether the patient had tuberculosis, they performed an exploratory operation to see if she was suffering from Hodgkin's disease.

The operation in fact revealed that she was suffering from tuberculosis. As a consequence of the operation, she suffered damage to the nerve affecting her vocal cords and consequently her speech was impaired. It was alleged that the consultants had been negligent in performing the operation before the result of the test for tuberculosis was known.

The evidence of an expert was that the patient had almost certainly been suffering from tuberculosis at the outset and this should have been diagnosed. It was wrong and dangerous to undertake the exploratory operation. The court said 'it is not enough to show that subsequent events show that the operation need never have been performed if at the time the decision to operate was taken, it was reasonable'.[11]

Differences of opinion in practice exist in the medical professions. There is seldom any one answer exclusive of all others to problems of professional judgement.

It would be unfair to health professionals to be deemed negligent where a decision had been made carefully and with great consideration, which is supported by a body of competent professional opinion, even where there is also a body of professional opinion that would not have followed that practice.

In practice this means that health professionals will be expected to follow acceptable standard procedures laid down by their professional bodies or the local policies of the employer. However, there may be very exceptional circumstances where it is justifiable not to follow the approved practice and the health professional must justify why they have not done so.

PROTOCOLS, POLICIES, PROCEDURES AND GUIDELINES

There are guidelines and codes of practice set down by professional bodies, regulatory bodies and at local level by the employer. Protocols, policies, procedures and guidelines are laid down for good reason. They provide health professionals with a safe framework for practice. They should be followed as far as is reasonable.

Whilst these codes of practice and guidelines are not legally binding, they are recommended practice. Breaches of them do not usually in themselves give rise to civil or criminal liability (except midwives under the NMC

Midwives' Rules[12]). However, a breach may be evidence of failure to follow the approved practice and it could be argued that such breach constituted negligence.

Indeed, the case of Cope v Bro Morgannwg NHS Trust 2005 illustrates that the failure to follow procedures in itself constituted negligence.[13]

CASE

Cope v Bro Morgannwg NHS Trust 2005
Mrs Cope contracted MRSA at hospital after a hip replacement operation in February 2001. The infection meant her new hip had to be removed. She took legal action against the Trust that ran the hospital, claiming it had allowed her to contract MRSA by failing to implement its policies and treat the infection appropriately. The hospital accepted it had not followed its own guidelines on infection control in her care.

The case was settled out of court.

This case illustrates that failing to follow the policy was negligent.

Following policies is no defence!

Health professionals are expected to follow policies and yet they may be alarmed to discover that following protocols and guidelines is not a defence if something goes wrong.

Protocols, policies, procedures and guidelines provide a framework for good and safe practice. However, such documents cannot be drafted to cover every eventuality. They should be applied to practice and not just blindly followed.

EXAMPLE OF BLINDLY FOLLOWING PROTOCOL

A patient is admitted into hospital for general surgery. He has a history of mental illness and is known to set fire to things. With this in mind the staff decided to move this patient to a single side ward outside the nurses' station so they can keep an eye on this patient. When moving the patient they transfer amongst his belongings a box of matches. That night the patient sets fire to his bedclothes, killing himself and injuring other patients and staff.

> The staff were asked 'Why did you leave the matches with the patient?' The reply was, 'The protocol states we are not allowed to interfere with the patient's belongings.'

Clearly this was not the intention of the protocol. A protocol cannot possibly be drafted to cover every eventuality. In this scenario the nursing staff will be accountable. It is not appropriate to blindly follow the protocol rather than critically applying it. They cannot hide behind the argument that they were following the protocol. This is not a defence.

Health professionals should follow these protocols and guidelines as far as is reasonable, but they should be critically applied and not blindly followed. A good record of how and why any procedure or policy has been departed from should be made. The health professional must justify their actions.

A failure to adhere to the guidelines or protocols or blindly following them, rather than critically applying them, may give rise to repercussions for breach of the professional code of conduct and may constitute a breach of duty of care.

Continuing responsibility for policies

A manager has a continuing responsibility to ensure that procedures, policies and guidelines are designed and implemented to prevent harm to the patient. If a health professional is aware of any problems with such policies they must report this to their manager. If there are shortcomings in such procedures, policies and guidelines, and no action is taken by health professionals or managers to rectify them, the health professionals will be seen as simply condoning poor practice. This will have repercussions for breach of professional code of conduct and is likely to constitute a breach of duty of care.

FAILURE BY MANAGERS TO ACT

'There's no point in telling management; they never do anything about it.'

A health professional is accountable if they fail to bring to the attention of their managers any potential harm or hazards to patients due to shortcomings in, for example, policies and guidelines or difficulties caused by staffing levels or lack of resources. Many health professionals complain that matters are being brought to the attention of the manager, but nothing is being done about it. However, it will not provide a defence to health professionals to say the reason you did not tell management is because they never act upon it.

The health professional has a duty to ensure that patients are cared for appropriately. If management does not act on concerns about potential harm to patients the health professional raising such concerns should express them in writing. A clear account should be provided, supported with facts. If the manager takes no further steps then the health professional must take it to the next level of management and proceed through to the chief executive if necessary. Managers who fail to deal with concerns raised may also be called to account by their professional bodies in respect of their fitness to practice.

BREAKDOWN IN COMMUNICATION

Breakdown in communication results in a vast majority of clinical accidents and legal claims, often through poor record keeping, system failures through lack of communication or poor verbal communication with patients.

As previously stated in its 2008 annual report, the NHSLA estimated that its total liabilities in outstanding clinical claims were £11.9 **billion**.[14] This includes the costs of compensation paid out and legal costs. It does not include the cost of staff and management time in dealing with those complaints, or the additional costs of bed space, so the true cost is far higher. The vast majority of clinical accidents arise as a result of a breakdown in communication through poor systems and poor documentation.

If a health professional fails to communicate adequately, either through poor records or in some other way, they will be accountable.

Health records

A patient's care is shared between a number of health professionals and the records provide an effective means of communication between them. If a health professional fails to maintain adequate records, and therefore does not communicate information to a colleague who then acted in a way that was detrimental to the patient, this would give rise to legal claim and would also constitute professional misconduct. In making a record, you should also be aware of the reliance which your professional colleagues will put upon it. Good communication is therefore essential.

Any delay in information reaching the records may result in a breakdown of communication. It is therefore essential for good risk management that all records are made contemporaneously. That is, they should be made at the same time.

Health professionals are responsible for maintaining a good standard of records. It is no defence that you did not have time to write them. You do not want to be in the witness box saying 'I am sorry the patient died but I did not have time to write the records.' The health professional will be accountable.

Verbal communication

CASE

Coles v Reading HMC 1963

The patient suffered a crush injury to his finger. He attended a local cottage hospital where the nurse cleaned the wound and told him to go to his doctor for an anti-tetanus injection. She did not impress upon him the purpose or importance of this so the patient did not go. The patient subsequently died of tetanus.[15]

In this case the nurse would be deemed to have been negligent.

Advice given to patients or other health professionals must be clear and unambiguous.

Telephone calls

Many cases will stand or fall on the basis of a telephone call that has not been relayed or recorded. Health professionals are often in the position where they are giving or receiving information and advice over the telephone, either with other health professionals or patients. In these circumstances, the health professional must ensure that the advice has been understood. It is good practice to repeat the instructions or advice back to the advisor. This will avoid any misunderstandings and will ensure that the patient will receive the correct treatment. A detailed note of the advice given or received must be made in the patient's record.

The following case illustrates the hazards of diagnosing over the telephone.

CASE

Hazards of diagnosing over the telephone

A child was born prematurely and developed hydrocephalus – an abnormal amount of cerebrospinal fluid around the brain. A tube was fitted to drain the excess fluid from his skull to avoid the build-up of excessive pressure within the brain. The child's condition was well documented within his GP records and he had experienced difficulties with the tube blocking on previous occasions, which had been acted upon quickly and treated.

The child complained of a headache and had vomited suddenly. His mother called the GP for advice and during a short telephone call the GP diagnosed a viral infection.

The following day his symptoms deteriorated and he was rushed to hospital where it was found that the tube in his skull was blocked. He suffered a cardiac arrest and the increased pressure in his skull had caused damage to his brain.

His mother's and the GP's recollection of their telephone conversation was quite different. This discussion was considered in some detail during the court trial, which addressed whether the GP had provided the child with a reasonable level of care. Many issues arose including how the child's mother actually described his symptoms. Should the GP have asked specific questions to rule out a blocked tube? Was a visit to the GP and/or a home visit mandatory and did the GP take a satisfactory medical history?

The judge in this case found that the GP was in breach of his duty of care to the child by failing to take a sufficient history to exclude the possibility of a blocked tube. It would have been common sense for the GP to ask specific questions to exclude a tube blockage and there was no logical basis for not asking these. If this had been done the child would have been referred to hospital a day earlier and his brain damage would have been prevented.[16]

A detailed record of the information obtained and advice given should have been made in the health records. The GP will have given advice to many patients during the course of his work and in the absence of an entry in the records the GP is unlikely to recall the details.

Faxes

A fax that has not reached the recipient can have devastating consequences. Health professionals must ensure that a fax they send has been received by the correct recipient. A simple telephone call will suffice.

CASE

Fax error

The Times, dated 16 December 1997, reported that a girl died because her medical records were faxed to a machine in a locked room to which no one had access over the weekend.

The girl was aged five years and suffered from giant cell hepatitis. She fell ill on a visit to Middlesbrough, where, in ignorance of her medical history, she was given a new drug, tacrolimus, and suffered a massive overdose.[17]

Health professionals must ensure that there can be no confusion or room for error and should not rely solely on a faxed document.

DUTY TO INFORM THE PATIENT OF A MISTAKE

If a health professional is aware that a mistake has been made and neither the patient nor the relatives have been informed, does the health professional have a duty to inform the patient?

A health professional has a duty to ensure that the patient receives treatment and care in accordance with acceptable standards of practice. If a mistake has been made by a health professional or their colleague in, for example, administering the wrong dose of drug, it is essential that the health professional makes this known so that appropriate treatment may be implemented. Health professionals should also take steps to ensure that such an error does not occur again. If a mistake has been made by a colleague then the health professional should complete a report. If the health professional themselves have made a mistake, they should report it as they have a professional duty to do so.

It is good practice to provide full disclosure to the patient. The health professional in charge of the patient's care is responsible to ensure that this is done and to reassure the patient about any effects. The health professional must take all reasonable steps to ensure that the patient is fully informed.

SYSTEM FAILURES

With changing dynamics of healthcare, reforms and regular reorganisation can result in confusion over roles and responsibilities for the delivery of care. Who is responsible when a patient is injured as a result of a system failure?

Much of what a health professional does from day to day is reliant upon efficient and effective systems. Patient data, appointments, records, IT, infection control, admissions, theatres, to name but a few, are all reliant upon appropriate systems. System failures often result from a breakdown in communication, poorly drafted or applied guidelines and an ignorance of the systems and procedures.

The London Ambulance Service (LAS) introduced a new computer-aided despatch system in 1992, which was intended to automate the system that despatched ambulances in response to calls from the public and the emergency services. This new system was extremely inefficient and ambulance response times increased markedly. Shortly after its introduction, the new system failed completely and the LAS reverted to the previous manual system. The system failure was not just due to technical issues, but to a failure to consider human and organisational factors in its design.

The computer system built to run NHS patient records experienced so many problems that there were concerns that patients could be put at risk. There were technical problems with missed appointments, lost records and lengthy delays for patients needing to see specialists.

Cleaning systems undertaken in some hospitals are ineffective resulting in patients contracting infections.

Poor systems for the packaging and labelling of medicines that look similar will increase mistakes being made in hospitals and pharmacies and can put lives at risk.

Since 1975 at least 13 patients in the UK have died or been paralysed as a result of being erroneously administered intrathecally instead of intravenously with the anti-cancer drug vincristine. A contributing factor for this error included premature removal of the drug from its over-wrap packaging.

CASE

Injection site error

In 2001, a teenager, Wayne Jowett, died as a result of an anti-cancer drug being accidentally injected into his spine instead of a vein. Staff had been reminded to follow strict protocols and procedures for administering such drugs to patients.[18]

It was recommended that a spinal syringe should be designed so it cannot physically be joined to an ampoule containing a drug that should not be given intrathecally. However, the design has still yet to be agreed.

Who is responsible?

If a patient is injured as a result of a system failure who bears the responsibility? It would be nice to reassure the health professional that a system failure is the responsibility of the employer. However, this is not necessarily the case. It will depend upon the circumstances of each situation.

EXAMPLE OF SYSTEM FAILURE

In an unreported case involving Mrs S, a 28-year-old woman was admitted for routine surgery for a prolapsed disc. She was the third patient on the theatre list. The first patient had been operated on and the instruments were being sterilised. The instruments were required for patient number two and rather than wait for the instruments to come out of the steriliser, the surgeon swapped the list around. Mrs S then became patient number two. Part-way through the procedure they realised they had forgotten to swap the blood bags over and had administered a wrong blood type transfusion. The patient died on the theatre table.

At the inquest the anaesthetist who had failed to check the wristband with the blood bag explained 'I am new to the Trust; I trained and worked abroad and we did things differently there.'

The surgeon said 'next time I swap the list around I will tell people'.

This is a classic example of a system failure and a breakdown in communication. The surgeon tells the theatre nurse, the nurse goes on his coffee break and tells someone else who tells someone else and so on. The original message is diluted and becomes 'Chinese whispers'. It results in a breakdown in communication – in this case with tragic consequences.

In this instance, the Trust would be responsible for paying compensation to the deceased's family. The surgeon and the anaesthetist will be accountable to the professional body and the employer. If their actions are deemed to be gross negligence they could even face criminal charges of manslaughter.

If a system is not effective, health professionals have a duty to bring this to the attention of management. Management have an ongoing responsibility to ensure that systems are safe and effective.

A national reporting system is currently being developed. A better understanding of the human factors involved in lapses, mistakes and protocol violations by medical professionals is also being pursued to aid design of safer ways of working.

WORKING LONG HOURS

Imagine being on an aircraft waiting to take off when an air steward makes an announcement: 'The pilot is rather tired today as he has just come off a long haul flight but there is no other pilot to take over the aircraft. I'm sure he will be fine'. How many passengers do you suppose will be happy to stay on the aircraft?!

The European Working Time Directive (EWTD) limits the number of hours per week employees should work. However, despite these rules, many health professionals work far in excess of them.[19]

Working long hours causes stress, illness and demoralises health professionals. Tiredness may result in lapses in concentration. There is a real danger that patient care will be compromised, particularly where care or the task requires a degree of skill.

TASK

What does a health professional do if they have finished their shift but the next shift rings in sick and it takes time to find a replacement?
- Do they leave the patients unattended?
- Or do they stay and put the patient at risk because they are tired?

Clearly the health professional should not leave patients unattended. If they do they will be accountable. They must make alternative arrangements for cover and management should be informed to deal with the situation.

If the health professional stays to assist and because they are tired something goes wrong, they will be accountable.

An employer cannot reassure a health professional who is expected to work long hours that if a patient is injured as a result of their tiredness, they will stand by them. Remember the areas of accountability. The employer cannot protect the health professional against criminal liability, or breach of professional conduct and cannot prevent the patient suing for compensation.

The health professional must have the skill, ability and competency to undertake the tasks. Tiredness may impact on this. If patient care is compromised as a result, the health professional will be accountable.

TEAM DECISIONS

'It was not my decision, it was a team decision'!

Healthcare is usually performed as part of a team. Very few tasks are performed entirely by one health professional. In the community, on a ward or during surgery all involve team care.

What is the situation when a decision about a patient is made by a team? Who is accountable? What if a member of the team does not agree with the decision? Are they still accountable?

The law does not recognise a team decision. Each member of that team will be accountable individually. To have a finding of team negligence would be very unfair as it presupposes that a student has the same knowledge as a consultant and that they are equally culpable.

A health professional cannot absolve themselves from responsibility by saying it 'was not my decision, it was a team decision'. You cannot use this as a defence.

CASE

Wilsher v Essex Area Health Authority

In this case a junior doctor working in a special care baby unit put a catheter into the wrong blood vessel which resulted in excess oxygen and the condition of retrolental fibroplasia; and the baby subsequently became blind. The doctor argued that this was an easy error to make in such a small infant and as he was a junior doctor you could not expect any more.

The court rejected this argument and held that junior doctors are required to adhere to the same standard of care as those who are more senior. The concept of 'team negligence' was considered, and it was held everyone working in the unit was expected to exercise the same professional standard, and to look to a more senior person for advice if necessary.[20]

EXAMPLE OF A TEAM DECISION

A young girl took an overdose and required a liver transplant, which was carried out. She needed a further transplant. The decision of the team was that no further transplant should be given.

The girl died and the family said that the second transplant should have been carried out and that it would have saved her life.

A doctor's evidence was that it was not his decision, it was a team decision.

The court does not accept this. It is your decision and you must justify it.

You must be able to say 'it was my decision', you can then go on to say 'and my colleagues were of the same opinion'. But you cannot say that you were bound by a higher order.

OBEYING ORDERS

'Don't be impertinent, don't question me, just do as I say.'

A health professional is often confronted with the situation of being told to do something, even though to do it may be against their better judgement. What is the position of the health professional when they are obeying orders?

The health professional will still be accountable for their actions notwithstanding that they have been ordered to carry those actions out. This is particularly difficult for junior staff who may not have the courage to say 'no' to their manager, their boss or a senior health professional.

TASK

A doctor writes up a prescription for a patient for a new drug that has just been released onto the market. The health professional on duty is not sure about the drug and says that he would like to check with the pharmacist before administering it. The doctor is very annoyed and says 'don't be impertinent; don't question me, just do as I say'.

What is the position of the health professional if he administers the drug?

The health professional must take all reasonable steps to ensure that the correct medication is being given, in the correct dose, in the correct way and at the correct time. If it is non-urgent the delay in seeking advice from the pharmacist would not have caused any harm to the patient.

If the health professional proceeded to administer the drug on the orders of the doctor and something went wrong resulting in the patient suffering harm or death, the health professional would be accountable. The health professional would be negligent in a civil claim, could face disciplinary action before the professional body and would be accountable to the employer.

It might be different if the situation was urgent. Acting in an emergency is discussed later in this chapter.

In any legal proceedings, the health professional would have to show that they acted reasonably having regard to approved and accepted practice.

The health professional cannot justify his actions and it is not a defence simply to say 'I did it because I was following orders.'

How to deal with orders in practice

A problem can arise where a health professional expresses their concern about carrying out an order but they are ignored. It is important not to put the patient at risk. Where the health professional fears that following an order could cause harm to a patient but their concerns are being ignored, the health professional should report it to their line manager and, if necessary, seek advice from a more senior doctor. This need not be confrontational but open discussions should be encouraged, perhaps including other members of the team.

A health professional should not disobey the orders of a superior lightly and there should be compelling reasons for doing so. A good record must be made of the order given, discussions and steps taken so that the health professional can justify their actions. If an order is unreasonably disobeyed then the health professional may face disciplinary action by their employer. If the patient is injured as a result of disobeying orders then the health professional may be liable in a civil claim and could face disciplinary action before the professional body.

ACTING IN AN EMERGENCY

Health professionals are often confronted with an emergency. They can be faced with very difficult situations, on a ward, in the community, during a major incident or in a war zone such as Iraq. Is the health professional accountable if something goes wrong in such circumstances?

Community care

TASK

A health visitor attends a patient who is very unwell. She suspects that the patient has an infection and he is having breathing difficulties. The health visitor telephones the GP who says he will visit the patient following his surgery. Immediately following the conversation with the GP the patient subsequently stops breathing. The health visitor attempts resuscitation during which she breaks several of his ribs. The resuscitation fails and the patient dies.

The family complain that his condition should have been treated as an emergency. They are very upset that during resuscitation the force used was unnecessary and that this caused the broken ribs. They say that calling the GP delayed his treatment and that if the health visitor had called an ambulance instead then the patient might have survived.

What is the liability of the health visitor?

The health visitor must act reasonably according to accepted practice. In these circumstances the health visitor will be expected to identify that the patient was unwell and to instigate appropriate care.

During the resuscitation procedure the health visitor broke several of the patient's ribs. It is not uncommon that ribs are broken during the procedure, particularly with the elderly. The health visitor was acting in an emergency to save the patient's life and this will be weighed against the risk of breaking the patient's ribs. The health visitor is likely to be seen as acting reasonably in these circumstances.

The health visitor realised that the patient was unwell and called the GP. This may have been appropriate depending on the specific signs and symptoms. For example, if the patient's condition was acute and the collapse could not have been anticipated then the health visitor may not have been expected to consider the situation more urgently and it was reasonable therefore to wait for the GP to call later.

However, if the health visitor realised or ought to have realised that the patient required urgent treatment, the health visitor will be accountable for not calling an ambulance.

The health visitor may be negligent giving rise to a civil claim, may face disciplinary proceedings before the professional body and may be accountable to the employer.

Major incident

In some situations acting in an emergency can be very difficult, for example, where there has been a major incident. A health professional may be called upon to assist and they may be faced with a situation that falls outside their expertise.

TASK

There has been a major train crash and 55 people have been seriously injured and are taken to hospital. It is 4:00 a.m. and there are very few staff on duty. Dr Jones, a junior doctor in oncology, has offered to assist the A&E department whilst they continue to try contacting more appropriately trained staff.

Dr Jones is faced with several patients. He makes an assessment as to which patients need more urgent care. Some are bleeding profusely, some are unconscious and some are walking wounded.

He sees a patient whom he does not consider to be seriously injured. The patient has a high temperature and low blood pressure. He administers antibiotics. However, Dr Jones fails to recognise the signs of internal bleeding and does not request a blood test. The patient is allergic to the antibiotics. The patient subsequently dies.

What is the liability of the junior doctor?

Organisations should have proper planning in place for major incidents to deal with emergency treatment, surgery and bed space. Appropriately trained staff will be called upon. However, it is not uncommon for health professional staff to make themselves available to assist until the arrival of more appropriately trained staff.

When dealing with an emergency it is difficult to obtain a patient history where the patient is incoherent or unconscious. The hospital may not hold any records for the patient and therefore there may be no indication that the patient may be allergic to antibiotics and that the patient may suffer a severe reaction. If, however, Dr Jones could have, but failed to take a history to establish any such allergic reactions, he will be accountable.

Dr Jones is an oncologist and so may not be expected to diagnose an internal bleed. However, he should have been able to identify that something was wrong and should have sought further advice and assistance. It may be that all other staff were dealing with medical emergencies, but Dr Jones must show that all reasonable steps were taken notwithstanding the emergency situation.

OBEYING ORDERS IN AN EMERGENCY

TASK

A patient suffers an acute collapse on a ward. A doctor places a cannula in the patient's arm and asks the health professional to set up the antibiotic for immediate intravenous infusion and hands the bag to the health professional. The health professional sets up the bag, but does not check the contents on its label. The patient deteriorates and dies. It is subsequently discovered that the content of the bag was something other than the antibiotic.

What is the position of the health professional?

The health professional should clearly have checked the label as this could have been done easily and would not have delayed the urgent treatment.

Notwithstanding the urgent nature of the situation, the health professional would be negligent in a civil claim, could face disciplinary action before the professional body and would be accountable to the employer.

The health professional cannot justify their actions by saying 'that was the bag I was given'. This is not a defence.

ON HOLIDAY

'I was on holiday at the time. It's nothing to do with me'.

Can a health professional be responsible for staff even when they are away on holiday when an incident occurs? The answer is yes!

Managers, supervisors and ward sisters, for example, who have responsibility, must ensure that the care of patients is carried out competently and diligently, even when they are absent. They must ensure that proper procedures and systems are in place. If they are not, managers, supervisors and ward sisters (i.e. those who should have implemented the procedures and systems) will be accountable.

OFF DUTY

Does a health professional have an obligation to care for a patient when they are off duty? It is not uncommon for health professionals to be expected to become involved in patient care when they are off duty. This is particularly common in community care.

TASK

Sandra, a health visitor, is off duty. She is shopping in the supermarket on Saturday morning with her family when one of her patients approaches her and says 'Look at my baby, don't you think he's looking a little peaky today? Should I be worried about him?'

Does Sandra have an obligation to check the baby?

If Sandra does not check and the baby deteriorates, will Sandra be accountable?

Whether Sandra has a legal obligation can be difficult to determine. In practice, however, it is often quite difficult for a health visitor in such immediate circumstances to ignore the concerns of the mother.

Whether Sandra will be liable if something were to happen to the baby will depend upon the way she may be deemed to be negligent. For example, if there were clear and obvious signs, such as a rash that showed the baby was at the time suffering from meningitis, and Sandra failed to act upon it then she may indeed be liable.

However, it would be impractical to carry out a thorough examination in the supermarket, and if there were no obvious signs Sandra could not be expected to determine that the baby was so unwell. In the circumstances Sandra may not be negligent. It would have been appropriate to advise the mother to seek advice from the GP if she was worried about the baby. If Sandra failed to do this she may be guilty of professional misconduct.

EXAMPLE OF PROFESSIONAL MISCONDUCT

A nurse who came before the conduct committee was found guilty of misconduct when she refused to answer a heart patient's call for help because she was having her tea break.

This was later appealed successfully at the Court of Appeal because it had not been established that the nurse knew it was an emergency.

However, if the matter had come before a civil court in a claim for compensation, different principles apply and the nurse may indeed have been deemed negligent.

This situation is different from the 'Good Samaritan rule', which is discussed in Chapter 17.

REFERENCES

1 Mental Health Act 1983.
2 Care Standards Act 2000.
3 Nursing and Midwifery Council. *NMC A-Z Advice Sheets*. London: NMC.
4 Crawford v Charing Cross Hospital. *The Times*. 8 Dec 1953.
5 Bolam v Friern Barnet 1957 2 All ER 118.
6 Nettleship v Western 1971 3 All ER 581.
7 Jones v Manchester Corporation 1952 2 All ER 125, (CA).
8 Edward Wong Finance Company Ltd v Johnson Stokes and Masters 1984 AC 296.
9 MV Herald of Free Enterprise: Report of the Court No. 8074 (1987).
10 Bolitho v City and Hackney Health Authority 1997 3 WLR 115.
11 Maynard v West Midlands Regional Health Authority 1985 1 All ER 635; 1984 1 WLR 634.
12 Nursing and Midwifery Council. *Midwives' Rules and Standards*. London: NMC; 2004. Available at: www.nmc-uk.org/aFrameDisplay.aspx?DocumentID=169 (accessed 29 March 2009).
13 Cope v Bro Morgannwg NHS Trust 2005. Available at: http://mrsaactionuk.net/2009AGM.html (accessed 20 April 2009).

14 National Health Service Litigation Authority. *Report and Accounts: fact sheet 2, financial information*. London: National Health Service Litigation Authority; 2008.

15 Coles v Reading HMC 1963 107 SJ 115.

16 Gray N. The hazards of diagnosing over the telephone. Available at: http://alexanderharris. co.uk/article/The_hazards_of_diagnosing_over_the_telephone_2343.asp (accessed 20 April 2009).

17 News in Brief. Girl died after fax error at hospital. *The Times*. 16 Dec 1997.

18 Laville S, Hall C, McIlroy AJ. Wayne Jowett. *The Telegraph*. 19 June 2001.

19 European Union. *The Working Time Directive of the European Union – Council Directive No. 93/104/EC*; 23 November 1993. Available at: www.incomesdata.co.uk/information/ worktimedirective.htm (accessed 29 March 2009).

20 Wilsher v Essex Area Health Authority [1988] AC 1074.

CHAPTER 12

Lack of resources

Lack of resources or lack of facilities is never a defence to a claim for negligence. This may seem harsh when often resources can be outside the control of many health professionals.

Where a patient is injured as a result of lack of resources and the patient sues, the organisation will pay out the compensation because of vicarious liability (*see* Chapter 2). The individual health professionals will also be accountable.

DUTY OF LOCAL AUTHORITY

Care in the community, which is managed by social services, is subject to the National Assistance Act 1948.[1] This Act makes it compulsory for the local authority to, for example, provide equipment or care where the need has been identified. This is a statutory duty and they must obey it. If they fail to provide for the patient then the local authority will be in breach of their statutory duty. Due to the different obligations placed on the local authorities, the Trust and PCTs, there is often a struggle as to who should have the responsibility and with it the financial burden.

OBLIGATIONS ON HOSPITALS AND PCTs

The law relating to hospitals and PCTs differs from that which applies to local authorities. The law recognises that resources in healthcare are not infinite. The NHS is protected by 'reasonable provisions'. The NHS must make reasonable provisions with the available resources. You cannot expect every NHS body to meet patients' needs; however, once you accept a patient then you must deal with that patient appropriately.

CASE

Reasonable provisions

A child was suffering from maesthenia gravis and was likely to die before surgery could be offered. The parents brought the matter before the court to obtain an order that the hospital provide surgery more quickly to prevent the child from dying.

The judge said, 'Very sorry, but you cannot use the legal system to move up the waiting list – the Trust made a reasonable decision within the resources it had. It is not for the court to make those decisions.'

Once the care of a patient has been accepted, the patient must be looked after and resources must be made available to provide a reasonable standard of care.

It may be an issue for management if they accept a patient when the appropriate resources are not available. Management must assess the risk.

It should be noted that all health professionals have an obligation to bring matters of lack of resources to the attention of management. If they fail to do so they will accountable.

SCENARIO

At the A&E department of the hospital there is only one doctor on duty. It is Saturday night and the department is extremely busy. The waiting time is four hours.

A man is brought in from work with chest pains. He is seen and assessed by the triage nurse and is given a red tag thus requiring immediate treatment. There is no trolley in the department and the patient is told to go and sit down in the waiting area.

Three hours later they call his name. There is no response – the patient is dead in the chair.

A patient is entitled to an acceptable standard of care. Even in an emergency situation staff will be expected to prioritise appropriately to avoid harm to a patient arising.

Patients are vulnerable. The hospital cannot accept a patient and then fail to treat them. You cannot say 'come in, we will look after you' and then fail to treat them.

In the scenario above the hospital would be liable. The managers would also be liable in a claim for negligence and would also be accountable to their professional body and their employer. Health professionals must be proactive in dealing with lack of resources. You cannot sit back knowing such lack of resources is likely to result in harm to a patient. You will simply be condoning poor practice and for this you will be accountable.

Resources, whilst not infinite, must be managed reasonably.

SCENARIO

A patient is assessed as requiring three hours of physiotherapy a week. However, the Trust could only offer three hours a month due to lack of resources.

The patient sued the Trust because the patient failed to provide the three hours of physiotherapy a week the patient needed.

The Trust agreed that the needs had not been met.

Once a patient is admitted they are owed a duty of care. If the Trust cannot meet the needs then the Trust may be negligent.

If it is not possible to obtain sufficient numbers of staff or to run a service safely with the correct skill mix, then the provision of that service may have to be transferred to other providers.

LACK OF FUNDING

In the current poor financial climate faced by the health service there is a temptation to reduce costs by cutting back on staff and reducing beds. Cost cutting presents potential dangers to patients.

CASE

Cost cutting

In April 2007 it was reported that a PCT had been accused of approaching 'criminal negligence' over plans for reducing hospital admissions by cutting back on staff and bed space.

Doctors were concerned that there may not be enough beds for emergency patients with non-life-threatening conditions and they may have to be turned away.[2]

This would place extra burdens on GPs and the ambulance services.

Financial cut backs must be managed responsibly so the patients are not put at risk.

CUTBACKS IN TRAINING

There have been great criticisms over cutting back on training. Lack of training has a large impact on the overall resources available. If health professionals do not receive training they cannot undertake further tasks or accept expanding responsibilities. If they are not trained, they will not be competent. This is a waste of resources. The importance of training and regular updating cannot be overemphasised.

PRESSURES ON MANAGERS AND STAFF

Pressure on managers

Health professional managers are responsible for ensuring that resources are effectively used and are sufficient for treating patients according to the approved standard of care. If harm is caused due to inadequate resources and the manager fails to take appropriate steps to prevent unreasonable risk arising, then the managers will be accountable.

Understaffed

A problem often faced by health professionals and their managers is being understaffed. Harm to a patient may occur due to a shortage of staff. In court I have often heard it said that there were 'no funds available for agency staff', or 'agency staff who are not familiar with procedure require too much supervision which was too time consuming for short periods of cover'.

These excuses cannot be relied upon as a defence if something goes wrong due to a shortage of staff and the patient is harmed.

There are certain recommended staffing ratios set down by various researchers, but there is nothing specifically laid down in law regarding minimum staffing levels. The principles relating to liability in negligence will apply depending on the specific circumstances in each case.

A health professional has a duty to bring to the attention of their supervisors or managers any difficulties created by staffing levels to avoid risk of any harm to the patient. An inadequate number of trained staff in proportion to the needs of the patients could result in inexperienced health professionals acting outside their skill, ability and competency. In these circumstances, errors can occur in inexperienced staff administering wrong drugs or doses or erroneously using specialist equipment. Managers must ensure that senior management is notified of any dangers or hazards relating to staffing levels. A good record must be maintained of any such notifications.

TASK

Josie is a health visitor. She has been informed by her manager that two members of staff are off sick and it is not known when they will return to work. Their case load has been shared among the remaining heath visitors. Josie has been given so many cases that she cannot get around all of the clients. She is worried that she may not get to see them all and this could put them at risk.

What should Josie do?

Josie should prioritise her patients and ensure she is using her time appropriately. She should consider delegating some tasks to, for example, healthcare assistants. Josie should make sure her manager is aware that she has too many cases and the manager should then reallocate the care appropriately. The manager may need to get agency staff to assist. A good record must be made of all discussions and decisions and the rationale behind them.

Often health professionals do not want to make a fuss and will simply take what is thrown at them. By nature they are often very willing and as their primary consideration is the patient they will roll their sleeves up and get on with it. They often accept without question that there is no one else to undertake the extra burden, sometimes compounded by the fact that they are told by the manger 'there is no one else; we do not have the money for agency staff'.

If Josie was to take on too many patients and something went wrong, Josie would be accountable notwithstanding she did it with the best intentions. The manager will also be accountable if she does not deal with Josie's concerns appropriately.

TASK

Megan is a nurse manager. She has been informed by the staff that they have two empty beds, but they are so short-staffed due to holiday and illness the staff cannot cope and fear that if the beds are filled it will place the patients at risk.

What should Megan do?

Megan should ensure that all of the health professionals are using their time appropriately, that there is effective delegation and that tasks are prioritised, concentrating on the most important ones and not wasting time on those that can be safely left. If it is a critical situation then Megan should consider transferring staff from another ward or getting in agency staff. She will also need to consider whether they can cope with any further intake and, if not, make arrangements for other hospitals to take over admissions or transfer of patients. Waiting lists may have to be cancelled. A good record must be made of all discussions and decisions and the rationale behind them.

TASK

Joan, a midwife, was working on night duty. It was a busy shift. The supervisor asked Joan to take over the care of Lucy, who was in well-established labour. The supervisor was unable to give Joan a proper handover for Lucy.

Joan attached the cardiotochograph (CTG) monitor, but unfortunately the tocograph of this monitor did not work. Joan said the maternity unit was very busy so there was no one available to get her a replacement.

Joan had every intention to rectify this problem but events took over and she did not get a chance to sort it out.

Joan observed a prolonged period of bradycardia, but did not call anyone because there was no one free to assist her.

Eventually the supervisor came to assist because Joan had very recently returned to midwifery practice after a four-year break, and needed her expertise. The supervisor called the doctor who was in theatre and could not come immediately.

There was a delay in the delivery and the baby suffered hypoxia resulting in cerebral palsy.

Joan said they did the best they could in this difficult situation, given the lack of staff and medical support available to them at the time.

It could be argued that this incident took place because there was an inadequate level of staff. However, many factors must be taken into account. Were they so short-staffed that it would have been impossible for another member of staff to have helped Joan? Priorities should have been set. Joan had recently returned to work after a four-year break and therefore she should have been adequately supervised. Joan herself should also have taken steps to seek supervision and assistance in this situation. The supervisor was or ought to have been aware of the difficulties with staffing levels. It is reasonably foreseeable in the circumstances that such an incident may occur and Joan and the supervisor will be accountable.

Covering more than one ward

Many health professionals are concerned about the responsibility of covering more than one ward. After all, they cannot be in two places at once. Who is responsible if something were to go wrong when the health professional is absent?

A ward sister may hold the keys to the drug cupboard of another ward because there is no other qualified member of staff on that ward. In the circumstances, the ward sister will have the same responsibility for both wards. The ward sister must ensure that appropriate delegation and supervision is in place. If something were to go wrong due to, for example, lack of supervision, the ward sister would be liable.

REFERENCES

1 The National Assistance Act 1948.
2 Channel 4. *Despatches – Health*. Broadcast 26 April 2007.

CHAPTER 13

Delegating and supervising

DELEGATING

There is a change in the dynamics of healthcare provisions and more work is now being undertaken by healthcare assistants and support workers. Delegation is an area of concern to most health professionals. In particular there is a concern when delegating to non-regulated health professionals. It has become a daily task for health professionals to delegate to staff under their supervision.

Those being supervised may be healthcare assistants, trainees, volunteers or qualified staff. Healthcare assistants, for example, are now carrying out duties that were usually those of the nurses, such as assisting the patient to the bathroom and changing dressings or pads. Whilst the healthcare assistant is capable of carrying out these tasks, they do not have the skills, knowledge or expertise of the nurse. When changing pads, the nurse will not simply change a pad but will look for pressure sores and signs of infection.

Health professionals responsible for delegating tasks must ensure that those undertaking the tasks have the knowledge, skills and experience to carry out the task safely, effectively and are adequately trained. They must ensure the tasks allocated are appropriate to the individuals and adequate supervision is provided. If they are not health professionals, you must not ask them to do the work of health professionals. If they are training to be health professionals, you should be sure that they are capable of carrying out the task safely and effectively. If they are health professionals, you must not ask them to do work that is outside their scope of practice.

Whoever you ask to carry out a task, you must always continue to give adequate and appropriate supervision and you will remain responsible for the outcome.

If someone tells you that they are unwilling to carry out a task because they do not think they are capable of doing so safely and effectively, you must not force them to carry out the task. If their refusal raises disciplinary or training issues, you must deal with that separately, but you should not endanger the safety of the patient.

It is essential that those delegating care duties, and those employees undertaking delegated duties, do so within a robust local employment policy framework to protect the public and support safe practice.

The assessment, planning and evaluation of the patient's care must be documented. The health professional has a responsibility to ensure that any aspect of care delegated has been documented appropriately.

The records

Before delegation occurs, the health professional who is delegating the task must consider the following:

➤ the condition of the patient
➤ the competence of the person to whom the task is being delegated (there should be records to support and evidence this)
➤ how frequently the patient should be reassessed by the health professional regarding the continued delegation of the aspect of care, and
➤ the ongoing support arrangements that will be provided to those undertaking delegated duties.

Documentation should clearly outline any decision-making processes and must be patient-specific. The most appropriate place to record this information should be decided based on the working environment (that is, patient held records and care plans). At the point of each delegation, the names of those being delegated to must be clearly stated.

Accountability and responsibility for delegating

The health professional who delegates to another remains accountable for the appropriateness of that delegation and for ensuring that the tasks have been undertaken competently in order to promote optimum health outcomes for the patient. They will be held accountable for the actions of the person carrying out that delegated task. Health professionals are accountable for ensuring continued assessment of the competence of those to whom they are delegating.

If they fail to leave instructions when they should have done, their fitness to practice may be called into question and they will be accountable to their professional body.

The health professional carrying out the task may also be accountable, if, for example, they do not have the skill and ability to carry out that task and they fail to tell the person delegating about this, and something goes wrong.

Principles of delegation

All health professionals should have regard to the following principles and apply them in their own areas as a good practice guide.

➤ The delegation of care must always take place in the best interests of the patient and the decision to delegate must always be based on an assessment of the individual patient's needs.

➤ Where a health professional has authority to delegate tasks to another, they retain responsibility and accountability for that delegation.

➤ A health professional should only delegate an aspect of care to a person whom they deem competent to perform the task. And they should assure themselves that the person to whom they have delegated fully understands the nature of the delegated task and what is required of them.

➤ Where someone else, such as an employer, has the authority to delegate an aspect of care, the employer usually becomes accountable for that delegation. The health professional will, however, continue to carry responsibility to intervene if they feel that the proposed delegation is inappropriate or unsafe.

➤ The decision of whether or not to delegate an aspect of care and to transfer and/or to rescind delegation is the responsibility of the health professional and is based on their professional judgement.

➤ The health professional should refuse to delegate if they believe that it would be unsafe to do so or are unable to provide or ensure adequate supervision.

➤ It is essential that those delegating care, and those employees undertaking delegated duties, do so within a robust local employment policy framework to protect the public and support safe practice.

➤ Healthcare can sometimes be unpredictable. It is important that the person to whom aspects of care are being delegated, understands their limitations and when not to proceed should the circumstances within which the task has been delegated change.

➤ No one should feel pressurised into either delegating, or accepting a delegated task. In such circumstances, advice should be sought, in the first instance, from the line manager and then, if necessary, from their professional body.

Health professionals should have regard to their code of professional conduct when delegating.

SUPERVISING

Supervision enables health professionals to develop knowledge and competence, assume responsibility for their own practice and improve patient care.

It enables the health professional being supervised to identify solutions to problems, increase their understanding of professional issues, improve standards of patient care, further develop their skills and knowledge and enhance their understanding of their own practice.

Health professionals should have access to clinical supervision and each supervisor should supervise a realistic number of practitioners.

Preparation for supervisors should be flexible and sensitive to local circumstances.

Evaluation of clinical supervision is needed to assess how it influences care and practice standards. Evaluation systems should be determined locally and local policies should be reviewed and updated regularly.

Countersigning the records

Countersigning the records might be required by health professionals in certain circumstances where, for example, members of staff are being supervised, such as students or healthcare assistants. In these circumstances the supervisor might countersign the records. The purpose of countersigning is to ensure that the supervisor is content that the treatment and care carried out has been competently done. It does not necessarily indicate that the supervisor has witnessed the care carried out.

Countersigning gives the supervisor the opportunity to satisfy himself that the care was appropriate and to clarify any issues the entries raise. The supervisor may wish to add to the records where clarification is needed. The signatory and anyone who countersigns the records may be required to give evidence in respect of these records.

You should confirm at local level what is required when authenticating and countersigning the records.

CHAPTER 14

Waiting lists

Who is responsible when a patient is on a waiting list? How long can a patient be left waiting? Who is responsible when a patient is referred for care or treatment?

Letters of referrals may be sent by GPs, consultants or social services, for example, or they may be internal referrals. Who is responsible for the patient and at what point do they become responsible?

TASK

A physiotherapist at a hospital receives a referral letter from a GP. The patient is sent an appointment.
   Who is now responsible for the patient – the GP or the hospital?
   At what point is the hospital responsible?
- The moment the referral letter is received?
- When an appointment has been made?
- When the patient has been seen and assessed?
- When it is agreed that the hospital will treat the patient?

EXCESSIVE WAITING TIME

The Department of Health has set down targets in various areas to reduce waiting times.[1] There is no legal requirement to attend a patient within a specific time frame. A patient who considers they have waited too long would need to pursue the internal complaints procedure. However, circumstances could arise where an excessive waiting time may constitute a breach of a duty of care. This might arise in circumstances where a delay in treatment has exacerbated the patient's condition and is related to a failure to recognise the urgent nature of the patient's treatment. Referral pathways should be in place.

Many cases have been brought where patients have waited a considerable period of time for operations or other treatment. As discussed previously, the courts generally take the view that it is not for them to become involved in issues relating to resource allocation. However, in a recent case the court concluded that where the patients have waited for a significantly long period of time then the NHS should pay for the patient to have treatment abroad.[2]

The responsibility for patients on the waiting list will depend upon the specific situations.

1 Where treatment has commenced, responsibility for the patient is that of the care providers. The treatment and care must be carried out according to acceptable and approved standards of practice.
2 Where treatment has not commenced and the patient is on a waiting list, even though the patient's condition may deteriorate, the patient cannot bring a claim.
3 If it is deemed the patient has waited an unreasonable length of time for treatment, the NHS may be obliged to pay for the treatment abroad.

EXAMPLE OF LONG WAITING TIME

A GP refers a patient who needs a hip replacement to an orthopaedic surgeon for review.

The consultant sees and assesses the patient and informs the GP. 'Thank you for sending this patient, I agree with your assessment and agree that he needs a hip replacement. I have placed him on the waiting list and will see him in two years' time.'

There is no responsibility on the part of the consultant even if the patient's hip deteriorates. The responsibility is that of the GP's. The GP must refer somewhere else if it is considered that the patient requires more urgent treatment.

It is extremely important for health professionals to ensure that referrers are kept informed. This will enable the referrer to keep the patient under review or seek the services of another provider.

INADVERTENTLY CREATING A RELATIONSHIP

A health professional does not create a legal responsibility merely by assessing a patient. During the course of an assessment they may give general verbal advice or provide the patient with a leaflet. However, the health professional may inadvertently become responsible in the course of an assessment if they give detailed advice and support and the patient relies upon it to their detriment. In these circumstances the health professional will then become accountable.

EXAMPLE OF INADVERTENT RELATIONSHIP

Using the example above, a GP refers a patient who needs a hip replacement to an orthopaedic surgeon for review. The consultant sees and assesses the patient. He advises the patient that he needs a hip replacement, but there is a two-year waiting list. He tells the patient, 'In the meantime take analgesic if you are in pain and exercise your hip by walking as much as possible.' The consultant informs the GP. 'Thank you for sending this patient; I agree with your assessment and agree that he needs a hip replacement. I have placed him on the waiting list and will see him in two years' time.'

   If the patient in exercising exacerbates his hip problem the consultant will be accountable.

It would be wise not to keep a patient's case open. The patient should be discharged and placed on the waiting list and the referrer should be informed.

REFERENCES

1 Department of Health. *Hospital Waiting Times and Waiting Lists*. London: DoH; 2009. Available at: www.dh.gov.uk/en/Publicationsandstatistics/Statistics/Performancedataandstatistics/HospitalWaitingTimesandListStatistics/index.htm (accessed 21 April 2009).
2 Watts v Bedford Primary Care Trust 2003 EWHC 2184.

CHAPTER 15

Gifts and hospitality

There are restrictions on what health professionals can ask for or accept as gifts.

You may be offered gifts, favours or hospitality from patients or clients during the course of, or after a period of care or treatment.

The NMC Code of Professional Conduct (called 'The Code') states:

> You must refuse any gift, favours or hospitality that might be interpreted as an attempt to obtain preferential treatment.[1]

Health professionals can receive gifts or favours from a patient, but must be confident that the giving of these gifts could not be interpreted as being in return for preferential treatment. Health professionals are also reminded, when deciding whether or not to accept a gift or favour, to consult local policy. Failure to do so could result in the health professional being in breach of their contract of employment.

Similarly the GMC Good Medical Practice 2006[2] states doctors:

> must not encourage patients to give, lend or bequeath money or gifts that will directly or indirectly benefit you . . . you must act in your patients' best interests when making referrals and when providing or arranging treatment or care. You must not ask for or accept any inducement, gift or hospitality which may affect or be seen to affect the way you prescribe for, treat or refer patients. You must not offer such inducements to colleagues.

There are legal restrictions on the activities that pharmaceutical companies can undertake to promote medicines. These restrictions are set out in the Medicines (Advertising) Regulations 1994.[3]

A pharmacist who accepts inappropriate or expensive gifts may be considered to be in breach of the Medicines (Advertising) Regulations 1994.[4] In addition, the Royal Pharmaceutical Society's revised Code of Ethics, implemented on 1 August 2007, states that:

> Pharmacists must not ask for or accept any gift, financial reward or inducement that may affect, or be perceived to affect, their professional judgement.[5]

Pharmaceutical companies can only offer gifts that are inexpensive and relevant to the practice of medicine or pharmacy. Examples include stationery items (pens, Post-it notes, etc.), relevant books or software and clinical items (peak flow meters or tissues). Items for personal benefit are prohibited.

Pharmaceutical companies can provide medical and educational goods and services that enhance patient care or benefit the NHS and maintain patient care as long as the arrangements are not an inducement to prescribe, supply, administer, recommend, buy or sell any medicine.

Companies holding or sponsoring scientific meetings may offer appropriate hospitality to health professionals. However, the hospitality offered must not be excessive and must be limited to what is required to support the main purpose of the meeting and can only be provided for professional attendees. An example of inappropriate hospitality is where the invitation is extended to a spouse or partner who does not qualify to attend in their own right. It should be the educational programme that attracts delegates, not the hospitality or venue.

It is advisable to have local policies in place to deal with the giving and receiving of gifts.

REFERENCES

1 Nursing and Midwifery Council. *The Code: standards for conduct, performance and ethics for nurses and midwives. Gifts and gratuities.* London: NMC; 2008. Available at: www.nmc-uk.org/aDisplayDocument.aspx?documentID=4176 (accessed 20 April 2009).
2 www.gmc-uk.org/guidance/good_medical_practice/index.asp
3 Medicines (Advertising) Regulations 1994.

4 Ibid.
5 Royal Pharmaceutical Society. *Code of Ethics for Pharmacists and Pharmacy Technicians.* London: RPS; 2007. Available at: www.rpsgb.org/pdfs/coeppt.pdf (accessed 29 March 2009).

CHAPTER 16

Whistle-blowing

There is an obligation on all health professionals to bring any wrongdoing, hazard or danger to the attention of management.

In practice, health professionals have been concerned about the repercussions of reporting a colleague or manager. They may fear their career progression would be hampered. They may fear confrontation and the impact on their relationships that such reporting would have. Junior members of staff often find it particularly difficult to report senior members of staff.

Health professionals cannot turn a blind eye to issues that have been identified. If a health professional ignores wrongdoing, hazard or danger they are placing patients at risk. They will compromise patient care and the health professional will be accountable.

The Public Interest Disclosure Act 1998 (PIDA) was introduced to protect employees who are worried about wrongdoing in their place of work and want to 'blow the whistle'.[1]

A House of Commons press release commented that:

> A constant theme of recent major accidents, financial scandals, and episodes of abuse, from Maxwell to BCCI, from the Clapham Rail disaster to the Beverly Allitt case, is that someone inside the organisation realised early on that something was wrong but was afraid to speak out, or was afraid of being punished for doing so. Employers are entitled to loyalty and confidentiality in normal circumstances. But where there is serious malpractice, it is vital that people know that the law will protect them if they act responsibly. This is not just for their sakes – it will protect us all. If people are afraid to speak out when they

see something seriously wrong the abuse will continue and ultimately lives may be ruined.[2]

Several cases have highlighted the dangers of failing to bring wrongdoing to the attention of management. Enquiries into some of the worst frauds and disasters of recent years highlight the importance of acting early on concerns raised by employees.

Canoeing accident – In 1994, after four children drowned in a canoeing accident at Lyme Regis, the managing director of the centre was convicted of manslaughter and sent to prison for three years after ignoring a graphic warning. The court heard that two instructors had sent a letter to the chief executive of the centre a year before the accident, stating: 'You should have a careful look at your standards of safety, otherwise you might find yourselves trying to explain why someone's son or daughter will not be coming home.'

Cancer misdiagnosis – In 1993, 2000 bone tumour cases were re-examined after an inquiry discovered that a senior pathologist at Birmingham's Royal Orthopaedic Hospital had misdiagnosed 42 cancer cases. The inquiry found that two consultants had expressed doubts about the diagnoses over several years, but they failed to speak up through official channels.

Piper Alpha – In 1988, the Piper Alpha oil platform exploded 110 miles off the coast of Scotland. The death toll was 167. The inquiry found that 'workers did not want to put their continued employment in jeopardy through raising a safety issue that might embarrass management'.

Herald of Free Enterprise – In 1987, the ferry Herald of Free Enterprise capsized off Zeebrugge; 193 people died. The inquiry found that concerns about sailing with the bow doors open had been raised on five previous occasions. A suggestion had been made to fit lights to the bridge to indicate whether the doors had been closed. The inquiry concluded: 'If this sensible suggestion had received the serious consideration it deserved, this disaster may well have been prevented.'

CASE

Bristol Royal Infirmary – Kennedy Report[3]

This case involved complex heart surgery of babies between 1984 and 1995 where there was a high mortality rate. A public inquiry was set up in response to the anguish of the parents.

The GMC called the doctors into account and found that they should have realised the death rate was higher than in other hospitals and that they should have sent their small and very sick patients to units where they performed the operations better.

It was clear that many of the health professionals knew standards were not what they should be years before the scandal became public, but either shrugged off responsibility or hoped things would get better.

The anaesthetist 'blew the whistle' over the deaths of babies who might have been saved had they been treated elsewhere. His view was that the surgeons were just not good enough at complex surgery on tiny hearts. He realised that operations were taking longer than they should and raised his concerns with other doctors. His concerns were ignored. He informed 24 senior people of his worries, and yet nothing was done to stop the tragedy unfolding.

The anaesthetist said he had been threatened that he would not have a future at the hospital if he continued to question the death rates. He and his family moved to Australia as a direct result of the treatment he received after criticising the conduct of paediatric cardiac surgery. He believed no medical or non-medical professional in the NHS should have to endure the threats and discrimination that he had been subjected to.

This approach to whistle-blowing creates mistrust and encourages secrecy. The anaesthetist was doing the right thing for future patients.[4]

Health professionals feared victimisation for bringing any wrongdoing to the attention of management. The Kennedy Report, following the Bristol Inquiry, made a number of recommendations to ensure that health professionals should not be penalised for raising concerns. They recommended, amongst other things, that there should be openness and honesty.[5]

THE PUBLIC INTEREST DISCLOSURE ACT 1998

This Act was introduced to protect employees who are worried about wrongdoing in their place of work and want to 'blow the whistle'. The Act applies to all NHS employees and includes all self-employed NHS professionals (i.e. doctors, dentists, opticians, optometrists, and pharmacists).[6]

An employee will be protected from victimisation if they disclose the information in good faith.

An employee who is victimised or penalised for making a protected disclosure can bring an action for compensation against the employer at an employment tribunal.

To qualify for protection your disclosure must be made in good faith and the wrongdoing must involve:

➤ a crime or breach of legal obligation (regulatory, administrative or common law)
➤ miscarriage of justice
➤ danger to health and safety
➤ damage to the environment; and/or
➤ attempts to cover-up such malpractice.

Health professionals should feel able to raise concerns with their employer. Each NHS body should have its own policy and procedures for responding to your concerns. A disclosure to the Department of Health is also considered to be a disclosure to your employer if you work within the NHS.

As a whistle-blower you are acting as a witness and not a complainant. You only have to have reasonable suspicion and not irrefutable evidence to support your concerns.

If you do suspect wrongdoing there are various things you should do.

➤ **Make an immediate note of your concerns.** Note all relevant details, such as what was said, over the telephone or in other conversations, the date, time and the names of any parties involved.
➤ **Convey your suspicions to someone with the appropriate authority and experience.** Most NHS bodies have established policies and procedures for whistle-blowing and your personnel department or head of internal audit should be able to provide you with further details. You can also get help and advice from the Department of Health.
➤ **Deal with the matter promptly, if you feel your concerns are warranted.** Any delay may cause your organisation or patients to suffer further or increase the risk of harm.

There are things you should *not* do.

➤ **Do nothing.**

➤ **Be afraid of raising your concerns.** You must not suffer any recriminations from your employer as a result of voicing a reasonably held suspicion. Your organisation must treat any matter you raise sensitively and confidentially.

➤ **Approach or accuse any individuals directly.**

➤ **Try to investigate the matter yourself.** This is particularly important if your concern is about a crime or breach of legal obligation. There are special rules surrounding the gathering of evidence for use in criminal cases. Any attempt to gather evidence by people who are unfamiliar with these rules may destroy the case.

➤ **Convey your suspicions to anyone other than those with the proper authority.**

If a health professional feels they are unable to raise the issue with their employer advice can be sought from their professional body or they can contact Public Concern at Work.[7]

Managers may wish to contact the National Patient Safety Agency (NPSA),[8] which collects reports from across the country and initiates preventative measures, so that the whole country can learn from each case, and patient safety throughout the NHS will be improved every time. The NPSA has established a network of patient safety managers to provide support and advice to NHS organisations.

For concerns regarding social care of adult and children's services you should contact the Commission for Social Care Inspection (CSCI).[9]

If the concern is about fraud or corruption within the NHS, the Counter Fraud Service has a reporting line.[10]

If the concern relates to financial matters other than fraud and corruption; for example lawfulness of expenditure, you should contact the Audit Commission.[11]

REFERENCES

1 The Public Interest Disclosure Act 1998.
2 House of Commons. *Bill will protect people blowing the whistle on serious wrongdoing.* Press Release. London: House of Commons; 13 February 1996.
3 Bristol Royal Infirmary Inquiry – Kennedy Report. *Learning from Bristol: the report of the public inquiry into children's heart surgery at the Bristol Royal Infirmary 1984–1995. Command*

Paper 5207; 2001. Available at: www.bristol-inquiry.org.uk/final_report/index.htm (accessed 29 March 2009).

4 *The Guardian* 18 July 2001. Available at: www.guardian.co.uk/society/2001/jul/18/all (accessed 20 April 2009).

5 Bristol Royal Infirmary Inquiry, op. cit. Kennedy Report, Chapter 23: Respect and honesty.

6 Public Interest Disclosure Act 1998.

7 www.pcaw.co.uk

8 www.npsa.nhs.uk

9 www.csci.gov.uk

10 www.cfsms.nhs.uk

11 Audit Commission dedicated PIDA Whistleblowers' Hotline on 0845 052 2646. Further information is available at: www.audit-commission.gov.uk/complaints/whistleblowing.asp (accessed 20 April 2009).

CHAPTER 17

'Good Samaritan' duty to volunteer help

THE OBLIGATION TO STOP AND ASSIST

TASK

Is there an obligation on a health professional to stop and assist someone when they are off duty?

A nurse is on her way out on a Saturday evening when she sees a road traffic accident where a pedestrian has been knocked over by a car.

Does the nurse have an obligation to stop and assist?

If she does stop and assist and something goes wrong, will she be liable?

There is no legal obligation for a health professional to stop and assist. However, there is a professional obligation.

In this situation, the nurse does not have a legal duty to stop and care for the injured person. But if she does, she then takes on a legal duty to care for the person appropriately. In these circumstances, it is reasonable to expect her to care for the person to the best of her abilities, using her nursing knowledge and skills and within her own level of competence.

If, as a result of the care she provides, she injures the person, then she may be liable. The person may sue for compensation and the rules of breach of duty of care, the 'Bolam principle' will apply. In these circumstances the nurse would be personally liable as she is not acting in the course of her employment so there is no vicarious liability on the part of the employer.

In some European countries they have the 'good Samaritan rule' whereby if, for example, a bystander assists a drowning person, they cannot be sued if something goes wrong. There is no such protection in the UK so the nurse could be sued. It would therefore be wise to check to see if the indemnity insurance covers such acts under the good Samaritan duty.

A health professional might consider it far too risky to stop and assist, so why bother? Whilst there is no legal obligation to stop and assist, a health professional will usually have a professional obligation to do so under their code of conduct. Therefore if they fail to stop and assist they will be in breach of their professional code of conduct.

WHAT IS EXPECTED IF THEY STOP AND ASSIST?

A midwife assisting victims of a road traffic accident or a geriatric nurse assisting a woman giving birth on a bus: how far must they go to provide care?

The health professional must care for the person to the best of her abilities, using their professional knowledge and skills and within their own level of competence. Where a passenger on a bus goes into labour the geriatric nurse would not be expected to know how to deliver a baby. It would be reasonable to summon appropriate help. The midwife, however, would have a greater duty of care in these circumstances and would be expected assist to a greater degree until help arrives.

To recap, a health professional has no legal duty to stop and assist, but they may have a professional obligation to do so under their code of conduct. If they assist and get it wrong they can be sued. If they do not assist they will be in breach of their code of conduct.

CHAPTER 18

Legal implications

CONSENT

Before you can treat a patient, valid consent must be obtained. The person carrying out the treatment is responsible for obtaining valid consent although it can be delegated in limited circumstances.

Consent may be written, verbal or implied. Valid consent depends upon a number of issues, such as how old the patient is, are they a minor, did they have the relevant information including the risks, did they understand it, did they have capacity?

Consent may become invalid through many factors; for example, how much time passed after consent was given before treatment commenced? Was the time frame too long or too short? Was consent given under pressure? Consent may be refused or withdrawn by the patient.

A good record of the patient's decision of consent must be made and communicated to all members of the health and social care team. Care must be exercised when using standard forms to ensure that documentation reflects in detail, and not just in general terms, what the patient is consenting to.

Health professionals should be familiar with local policies on consent. If valid consent is not obtained the health professional will be accountable.

Consent is a complex area and the health professional should be fully conversant with it.

GIVING ADVICE

Most health professionals will give advice to patients. Any advice given may be relied upon by the patient. If the advice is to their detriment, the health professional will be accountable.

The same principles apply to giving advice as they do in exercising skill, as discussed previously. A health professional may be negligent if the advice given results in harm.

EXAMPLE OF ADVICE CAUSING HARM

A health visitor advises a patient to undergo a course of treatment. The patient has an underlying heart condition, which the health visitor does not take into account.

The patient agrees to the treatment and suffers a heart attack as a result.

The health visitor failed to take into account the patient's underlying heart condition when giving advice. The patient relied on the health visitor's advice and has now suffered harm. The health visitor is accountable. The patient may sue for compensation and the health visitor would be considered to have been negligent. The professional body may strike the health visitor off the register and the employer may commence disciplinary procedures and ultimately dismiss the health visitor.

The same principle applies to all health professionals.

REFERRALS

Patient referrals may pass between, for example, the GP, community care health professionals, acute Trusts, social services or emergency care practitioners. They may be interdepartmental referrals, such as an acute Trust referring a surgical patient to the physiotherapist. It is imperative when making or receiving referrals that the information is properly communicated.

When making referrals ensure that an appropriate level of information has been passed on otherwise something may be overlooked; this could compromise the patient's care.

You should have regard to other issues such as the dangers of faxing information as discussed in a previous chapter. You should take steps to ensure that the fax has been received.

When receiving a referral you may need to make further enquiries regarding the patient's condition or history. You may need to obtain full access to the records. It is not a defence to say, 'the GP did not give me all of the information', or, 'I did not have all of the records to hand', or, 'the A&E department did not give me the x-ray'.

EXAMPLE OF NECESSARY FURTHER ENQUIRIES

A GP makes a referral to a psychiatrist. In the letter of referral the GP states the patient is displaying signs of schizophrenia. The psychiatrist sees the patient and prescribes drugs for schizophrenia. It later emerges that the patient was suffering from a brain tumour and was left untreated for several months. The tumour has now grown considerably and the operation to remove it is now more risky and the chances of survival have been considerably reduced.

The psychiatrist said the reason it was not picked up was because the GP had already diagnosed the condition and the psychiatrist was just treating it.

Who do you think is at fault?

The GP made a referral to a specialist having identified that the patient was likely to be suffering from a mental disorder. The GP would not have the specialist expertise to identify that actual condition, hence the referral being made.

It is a matter for the psychiatrist to obtain all of the relevant information and to assess, diagnose and then treat the patient. The psychiatrist cannot hide behind the GP.

It is important to ensure letters of instructions are clear, but they must not mislead the recipient.

EXAMPLE OF MISLEADING INFORMATION

A health visitor sees a patient whom she believes has a cough. She sends a referral letter by fax to the GP. The health visitor fails to inform the GP that the patient is coughing up blood and is having breathing difficulties. As a result the GP does not prioritise the patient. The patient was suffering from pneumonia and due to the delay in treatment, the patient died.

The health visitor will be accountable for failing to pass all the relevant information to the GP.

EXAMPLE OF NOT OBTAINING ALL RELEVANT INFORMATION

A patient is referred by the A&E department to the physiotherapist. They do not provide the x-ray or the records. The records department say it will take four days to retrieve the records. The physiotherapist commences treatment. The patient had a fracture, which had been overlooked by the A&E department and the treatment given by the physiotherapist has exacerbated the injury.

It is not a defence for the physiotherapist to say they were not given the x-ray or they could not obtain the records. They should have obtained all of the relevant information before commencing treatment. This demonstrates the dangers of poor communication between referrers.

Keep the referrer informed

Always keep the referrer informed. You must ensure that any discharge of a patient has been communicated to the referrer. If a patient was not seen or was discharged for any reason, the referrer must be told so that they can make alternative arrangements. If you do not keep the referrer informed they will assume that the patient is being cared for.

A health professional who fails to keep the referrer informed will be accountable.

TAPE RECORDING

The Kennedy Report that followed the Bristol Royal Infirmary Inquiry[1] recommended there should be respect and honesty. Patients must be kept informed about their treatment or care, and communication must be improved, including the use of tape recording. Patients, should they so wish, can make a tape recording of discussions with healthcare professionals when the diagnosis, course of treatment or prognosis is being discussed.

It can sometimes be difficult for a patient to retain information given to them by health professionals. The information can be complex and a patient may wish to raise further questions arising from the information.

They may need time to consider the information to decide upon a course of treatment.

Patients often find a tape recording of a consultation very useful. They can re-listen to it at home, with their family if they so wish, so they can discuss it and make decisions about their care and treatment.

REFERENCE

1 Bristol Royal Infirmary Inquiry – Kennedy Report. *Learning from Bristol: the report of the public inquiry into children's heart surgery at the Bristol Royal Infirmary 1984–1995. Command Paper 5207;* 2001. Available at: www.bristol-inquiry.org.uk/final_report/index.htm (accessed 29 March 2009).

CHAPTER 19

The law and midwives

In recent years there has been an increase in legal claims relating to birth trauma cases. Compensation for such claims, where, for example, a child suffers cerebral palsy as result of hypoxia because of a delayed delivery, can be as much as £3 million to £5 million. The cost of these claims is high due to the level of care that is required.

A midwife can be accountable in many of the areas we have looked at. In addition, there are further rules that apply specifically to midwives. These rules[1] have been set down together with a code of practice[2] by the NMC. All midwives should be familiar with these rules and the code of practice.

The law relating to midwives makes it clear that it is an offence for a person, other than a midwife or doctor, to attend a woman in childbirth, except in an emergency or in supported recognised training. A person who contravenes this is committing a criminal offence.

Common problems encountered by midwives include, for instance, issues of consent, such as when the patient does not want a midwife present at the birth. Or when the patient does not wish to have pain relief and then during labour changes their mind. In this case does the patient have capacity to change their mind? If the patient refuses a caesarean section and such refusal is likely to result in the death of the unborn child, would the midwife have an obligation to save the unborn child regardless of the patient's consent? The law relating to consent has the effect that you cannot compel the patient to undergo treatment if they are a competent adult.

Consent is a complicated area and all midwives should be familiar with it.

TASK

Susan wishes to have a natural birth. She has made it clear to the community midwife she does not want to have a baby in hospital and would like her husband to deliver the baby. She refuses all antenatal care.
   What should the midwife do?

Some patients are keen not to receive antenatal care during pregnancy and wish to have a home birth without the assistance of a midwife. The patient can refuse treatment provided they are a competent adult. There is no action that can be taken to prevent this even if it is not clinically desirable. You cannot compel the patient to come into hospital.

However, it is an offence for someone other than a midwife or doctor to attend a woman in childbirth. Therefore if Susan's husband assists the delivery of the baby then he will be committing a criminal offence, unless he was acting in an emergency.

If a midwife is aware of a situation such as this, she should inform the mother and the husband of the law. A midwife should make a good record of the warning given in the notes. The midwife should also inform their supervisor.

Midwives should have regard to this when being assisted by those who are not qualified and are under the direction or personal supervision of a duly qualified midwife. The difficulty here is in ensuring that the midwife is aware when the baby is imminent.

If a midwife is obstructed by an aggressive partner, a midwife can call for the assistance of the police.

Another issue of consent concerning midwives is where a patient refuses a caesarean section, which may result in her own death or that of her unborn child. If the patient is a competent adult there is little the midwife can do. You cannot compel the patient to undergo a caesarean section.

LIABILITY TO THE UNBORN CHILD

If a child is injured as a result of harm caused *in utero*, once they are born, a child has the right to claim compensation from the person who caused the injury. This is set out under the Congenital Disabilities (Civil Liability) Act 1976.[3] Where, for example, due to the negligence of the midwife, a delay in delivery causes the child to suffer cerebral palsy, the child will be able to pursue a claim for compensation under this Act.

However, a child cannot pursue a claim against its own mother. Where a mother refuses treatment that results in harm of the child, the child cannot sue its own mother. There is one exception to this and that is where the mother was driving a motor vehicle and she knew or ought reasonably to have known that she was pregnant and failed to take care for the safety of the unborn child. This is a curious situation. In practice the child would pursue the mother's motor insurance company.

MIDWIFERY CASE STUDY

This case study involving midwifery care, highlights breach of duty of care; skill and ability; breakdown in communication through poor record keeping; and professional accountability.

The Professional Conduct Committee heard the case of a registered nurse and midwife, who was working as an 'F' Grade core midwife in a hospital environment. The practitioner faced three allegations including a failure to obtain medical assistance or to contact the senior midwife for a patient who had high risk factors; a failure to keep adequate records of care for the same patient, (particularly with regards to observations and fluid balance charts and medication records); and a failure to undertake the proper transfer of care to the oncoming midwife. The patient concerned had undergone an emergency caesarean section and her condition included continued heavy blood loss and a drop in blood pressure.

The circumstances of the case

The midwife was working full-time on mostly night duty in the hospital. On the particular night duty concerned a patient was admitted for post-maturity induction. The patient was at term plus 11 days and her care progressed to a caesarean section late in the evening on her second day after admission. The patient delivered a baby boy, weighing 10 lb 14 oz. An estimated blood loss from the mother of 800–1000 mL was recorded.

A second midwife, giving evidence, explained that she gave a personal handover to the midwife while taking the patient back from theatre to the ward. From that time onwards the midwife held the care of the patient. Another witness on nightshift duty gave evidence to the committee, that following the patient's return to the ward, the midwife first cleaned and restocked the theatre, which took a few hours. After completing these tasks the midwife then asked the second midwife to assist her in washing the mother. The second midwife commented that in her experience it was unusual to wait a few hours to wash someone after a caesarean section.

The second midwife described that the patient was at that point very pale, sleepy and still sitting in a pool of blood. She was given a vomit bowl as she said she felt sick.

The second midwife had concerns and checked the birth register in the office, which informed her that the patient had experienced a high blood loss in theatre. The witness questioned the midwife on the condition of the patient and commented that there was no urgency in anything the midwife said and that the midwife made no reference to any concern about the patient's condition.

The committee also heard evidence that the midwife failed to keep adequate records of the patient following her recovery in the delivery ward. Evidence was given that following the patient's caesarean section delivery the midwife should have provided continuity observation notes to be recorded quarter-hourly.

The witness told the committee that there were no entries on the postnatal card. This was raised as a concern by the witness as the patient had high risk factors, particularly her long labour, the large baby and her blood loss.

Decision on the facts

The Committee found all the facts of the charges proved. They stated that in relation to the first charge they had heard strong and credible evidence from a number of witnesses that the midwife failed to call for medical assistance or contact a senior midwife when Patient A's clinical condition was deteriorating. This was evidenced by a continued heavy blood loss *per vaginum*, a raised maternal pulse and a fall in blood pressure.

In relation to the second charge, the committee found a clear failure to document the patient's temperature, the maternal pulse rate and blood pressure at 5-minute intervals as required for the first 15 minutes after commencing a blood transfusion. They also found evidence that supported inadequate record keeping in relation to the frequency and times at which maternal observations of pulse and blood pressure were taken. They found entries wholly inadequate in that there were clear omissions of recorded input, output and blood loss. There was also a failure to balance Patient A's fluid input and output as required. In relation to the medication records, they found inconsistencies in the time and recordings of the medication in the maternal notes.

In relation to the third charge that the midwife failed to provide a proper transfer of care of the patient to the oncoming midwife, the committee said that they heard evidence supporting the allegation from a number of midwives, which they found to be credible.

Decision on misconduct

The committee found that all the facts proved amounted to professional misconduct. They found that the midwife's record keeping was such that it failed to provide adequate communication as to the condition of Patient A or the serious nature of her deteriorating health in respect of the appropriate decision making that was necessary.

The committee cited that in failing to communicate with the oncoming midwife, the safety and well-being of Patient A was put at risk. They found the midwife had blatantly disregarded her duty to work co-operatively with the wider healthcare team in the best interests of those in her care.

Background

The committee heard evidence as to the midwife's employment history and profile, including evidence that she had a previous disciplinary hearing for breaching the administration of medicines policy that resulted in an oral warning kept on her record for six months. No mitigation was put forward on behalf of the midwife.

Decision

The committee decided to remove the midwife's name from the register with immediate effect. Their reasons were that the standard of care provided to Patient A by the midwife fell well below the standard expected of a midwife on the NMC register. They felt that in caring for a vulnerable woman following a caesarean section, the midwife failed to act in accordance with the Midwives' Rules[4] and the Code of Professional Conduct[5] and therefore contributed to the serious deterioration in Patient A's clinical condition.

They also noted that the midwife had failed to accept responsibility for her own continued professional development, in that she did not update her knowledge and skills in relation to skills and drills. The committee felt that the public would be at significant risk if the midwife were to remain on the register.

Record keeping in midwifery care is paramount. The Nursing and Midwifery Council has set down guidelines for record keeping in midwifery care.[6] In addition, Rule 6 of the Midwives' Rules, which came into force on 1 August 2004, emphasises that the records relating to the care of women and babies are an essential aspect of practice to aid communication between the health professional, the women and others who are providing care. They demonstrate the standard of care provided.[7]

The records provide an accurate and contemporaneous account of the treatment, care and support of the patient. The patient's condition, when giving birth, can progress quickly and it is essential that the condition and care provided can be ascertained from the records immediately. Care will be shared amongst a number of health professionals in these circumstances such as midwives, obstetricians and paediatricians. They will need to make decisions about delivery, for example, whether to carry out a caesarean section. The records will be crucial to their decision making as they will need an accurate picture of the patient's and the unborn baby's progress and condition. If the records are not maintained accurately and contemporaneously the health of the patient and the unborn baby may be compromised.

Midwives should have particular regard to documentation specific to them, for example, the CTG and partogram.

Notwithstanding the high incidence of litigation, midwifery records should not be written defensively with the court in mind. They should be written for the benefit of treating, caring and supporting the mother and baby.

REFERENCES

1 Nursing and Midwifery Council. *Midwives' Rules and Standards*. London: NMC; 2004. Available at: www.nmc-uk.org/aDisplayDocument.aspx?documentID=169 (accessed 29 March 2009).

2 Nursing and Midwifery Council. *The Code: standards for conduct, performance and ethics for nurses and midwives*. London: NMC; 2008. Available at: www.nmc-uk.org/aDisplayDocument.aspx?documentID=3954 (accessed 29 March 2009).

3 Congenital Disabilities (Civil Liability) Act 1976.

4 Nursing and Midwifery Council. *Midwives' Rules and Standards*, op. cit.

5 Nursing and Midwifery Council. *The Code*, op. cit.

6 Nursing and Midwifery Council. *Guidelines for Records and Record Keeping*. London: NMC; 2007. Available at: www.nmc-uk.org/aDisplayDocument.aspx?documentID=4008 (accessed 29 March 2009).

7 Nursing and Midwifery Council. *Midwives' Rules and Standards*, op. cit.

CHAPTER 20

Allied health professionals

Allied health professionals, such as speech and language therapists, physiotherapists, occupational therapists, chiropodists, podiatrists, radiographers, paramedics, emergency care practitioners, counsellors and psychotherapists, are subject to the law in the same way as any other health professional. Their professional bodies, such as the Health Professions Council (HPC)[1] and British Association of Counsellors and Psychotherapists (BACP)[2] set down a code of professional conduct with which members must comply.

No health professional is immune from litigation. There has been an increase in litigation in recent years against allied health professionals. These cases often include claims against physiotherapists, for example, for failing to check x-rays or the records before commencing therapy, resulting in inappropriate treatment. Or they can include claims against radiographers for failing to report appropriately or a failure to undertake x-rays in an appropriate timescale. There have also been claims against speech and language therapists for failing to identify or make appropriate referrals for clinical problems and claims against chiropodists for a failure to identify or treat infections.

CASE

Failing to identify clinical problems
Mary was six years of age, did well at school and was particularly confident in the performing arts. She suffered regularly from tonsillitis and was referred by

her GP for a tonsillectomy. Following an assessment she underwent surgery for a tonsillectomy and an adenoidectomy. Following surgery she developed a speech impediment. At the six-week review the consultant informed her that the impediment would improve. Six months later the impediment was still present and the GP referred her to a speech and language therapist. Therapy continued for two years with no marked improvement. In the meantime, Mary was being bullied at school because of her impediment. Her confidence had diminished, she was no longer active in the performing arts and her schoolwork was badly affected. She became very withdrawn.

It was then discovered that Mary had a congenital cleft palate and that an adenoidectomy should never have been carried out.

The consultant was accountable for failing to identify the cleft palate and then carrying out the adenoidectomy. This fell below the reasonable standard of care expected.

The speech and language therapist was accountable for failing to refer Mary back to the consultant. Mary's speech had not returned despite having been reassured that it would by the consultant. The therapist ought to have considered if there was a clinical reason for her impediment.

If an allied health professional fails to provide a reasonable standard of care in accordance with acceptable practice, they will be accountable.

RADIOGRAPHY

Radiography

The radiographer is accountable in the same way as any other health professional. They owe a duty of care when undertaking and reporting on x-rays and scans. If the patient is injured as a result of, for example, a delay, inappropriate or wrong reporting of an x-ray, or if no valid consent is obtained, the radiographer will be accountable.

Referral for x-ray

There are regulations concerning the ordering of an x-ray under The Ionising Radiation (Medical Exposure) Regulations 2000,[3] and the Ionising Radiations Regulations 1999.[4]

The directive lays down basic measures for the health protection of individuals against the dangers of ionising radiation in relation to medical exposure and the duties of those responsible for administering ionising radiation. In addition, it regards the need to protect those undergoing medical exposure, whether as part of their own medical diagnosis or treatment, as part of occupational health surveillance, or in health screening voluntary participants in research or medico-legal procedures.

The health professional referrer (the person ordering the x-ray) must have the authority of their employers to refer the patient.

X-rays must not be carried out unless the exposure is justified and authorised. Health professionals must provide medical data to enable the radiographer to decide whether or not a patient should be exposed to x-rays. They must have the relevant training and competency to carry out this task.

Matters that have come before the Health Professions Council include:

➤ failure to answer promptly to a request for an x-ray
➤ missing x-rays
➤ lack of skill
➤ failure to complete accurate and reproducible ultrasound examinations
➤ failure to follow protocols
➤ failure to interpret examinations accurately
➤ failure to make accurate records.

AMBULANCE SERVICE

The same principles apply to health professionals working in the ambulance service as to any other any health professional.

Some issues that often concern ambulance crew are systems of triaging, working long hours and consent issues, for example, where patients who do not want to go to hospital are pressured into going by family members. Care needs to be taken during the despatch stage at the control centre to ensure that the right cases are allocated to the emergency care practitioners and that they are triaged appropriately to ensure the response time does not compromise the patient.

Triaging

The introduction of the emergency care practitioner (ECP) and the system of referring a patient directly to a GP is an efficient use of resources. However, appropriate triaging is essential. ECPs have reported that triaging is often inadequate and a patient referred as non-urgent may often require more urgent treatment that is not appreciated until the ECP is at the scene. They may then need to call an ambulance to transport the patient to A&E, thus causing further delay.

Communication

It is paramount that records are properly maintained. Lack of clarity in carbon copy records, continuation sheets or a combination of electronic and written records can all lead to a breakdown of communication, which can compromise the care of the patient.

Emergency planning

The ambulance service must have procedures in place for emergency planning in the event of a major incident. As well as the practical aspects of emergency planning regarding, for example, deployment of vehicles and staff, they must also have in place a good system of recording for the designated loggists. The role of the loggist is to attend with the commanders at meetings and to accurately log the details of discussions and outcomes to ensure the efficient and effective lines of communication.

It must be remembered that should there be a public inquiry, an inquest or civil or criminal proceedings as a result of the major emergency, the records, including the logs will be produced as evidence and the writer may be called to give oral evidence in respect of them.

EMERGENCY CARE PRACTITIONER

The role of the ECP is a relatively new role and carries great responsibility. The ECP mainly deals with non-urgent patients where it is not necessary to transport the patient to the A&E department of the local hospital by ambulance, but rather to make an assessment of the patient's condition, provide care and make an appropriate referral. This role is akin to that of the GP and great care must be taken to ensure that the patient's history, condition and appropriate care is carried through.

One of the difficulties that can arise is lack of information, usually because the patient's records are not available. Issues of record keeping and referrals, discussed in previous chapters, are paramount.

Common complaints and litigation arising out of this role can involve failure to identify all of the signs and symptoms and/or failure to make an appropriate referral.

Good documentation is paramount. The records must be clear and unambiguous. Some of the reported problems with the records include ambiguity of the standard forms. For example, 'consent obtained Y/N'. But consent for what? This is an ambiguous section of the form.

The role of the ECP involves diagnosing and taking the next appropriate steps to treat the patient at home or to make a referral. These tasks are akin to those usually performed by a GP. However, the GP has the advantage that they have had more detailed training in anatomy and physiology rather than simply diagnosis. The ECP will be accountable if the diagnosis is not accurate or there is a failure to refer appropriately. It is not a defence that they are not well trained in anatomy.

I had the benefit of spending time with some ECPs and was able to give guidance regarding their documentation. During the process I assisted by recording information such as BP and blood gases, which was otherwise diffi- cult for the ECP to recall afterwards, as at the time they would be preoccupied with the hands-on care. The ECP commented how useful it was to have a secretary or loggist to assist in making the records, particularly a lawyer, and that he hoped this would be provided to all ECPs in future! I doubt that this will be the case and whilst this highlights the difficulties in practice, the records are paramount and cannot be compromised.

REFERENCES

1 www.hpc-uk.org
2 www.bacp.co.uk
3 Office of Public Sector Information. *The Ionising Radiation (Medical Exposure) Regulations 2000: statutory instrument 2000 no. 1059.* London: OPSI; 2000. Available at: www.opsi.gov. uk/si/si2000/20001059.htm (accessed 29 March 2009).
4 Office of Public Sector Information. *The Ionising Radiation Regulations 1999: statutory instrument 1999 no. 3232.* London: OPSI; 1999. Available at: www.opsi.gov.uk/si/si1999/ 19993232.htm (accessed 29 March 2009).

CHAPTER 21

Outpatient departments and walk-in centres

OUTPATIENT DEPARTMENT

Matters affecting the outpatient department often involve excessive waiting times, poor communication through the records, verbal communication or system failures.

Confidentiality is another area of concern in the outpatient department. This includes scrolling names in neon lights in the waiting area, or the calling out of patients' names, or making assumptions that if a family member is present then the patient must have consented to disclosure of all information. These are potentially breaches of confidentiality. Health professionals must be familiar with the issues of confidentiality.

Many difficulties arising in outpatient departments involve a breakdown in communication, such as patients falling through the review system or referral system, missing or wrong patients' records or poor recording of diagnostic test results.

The RCN has published competencies for outpatient nurses.[1] The framework focuses on treatment and care interventions that are specific to nurses working in outpatient departments. It is structured around six core characteristics of outpatient nursing, including:

➤ short interaction time with service users in outpatient departments
➤ supporting the service user when the message is uncertain
➤ diverse specialist interventions
➤ healthcare and developmental needs of outpatient departments service users

➤ multi-skilled interventions and discharge planning – the interface between hospital and community and health promotion.

Although this framework is intended to have a stand-alone function, it should also be used in conjunction with other frameworks that focus on the core skills and competencies for all qualified nurses. In addition, the specific frameworks developed by specialist nurses can be used to support and enhance outpatient nursing practice.

WALK-IN CENTRE

Any information or advice given out at walk-in centres or NHS Direct may be relied upon by the patient. If the patient acts on it to their detriment, the health professional who gave that advice will be accountable. The case of Coles v Reading,[2] (*see* Chapter 11), illustrates the dangers of unclear instructions.

Health professionals working in these environments may need to refer the patient for diagnostic tests or advise that the patient seeks specialist advice. Health professionals must have appropriate training and be aware of the limits of their knowledge.

REFERENCES

1 Royal College of Nursing. *Competencies for Outpatient Nurses.* London: RCN. Available at: www.rcn.org.uk/development/communities/specialisms/outpatients (accessed 30 March 2009).
2 Coles v Reading HMC 1963 107 SJ 115.

CHAPTER 22

Medication and prescribing

THE LAW

The law in relation to prescribing has been through some changes in recent years with extended powers of prescribing to non-medical health professionals and the concept of supplementary prescribers. There are many health professionals with great ability and skill and it was considered appropriate to make good use of these skills by extending the powers to prescribe.[1]

TASK

How does the law affect health professionals when administering and prescribing medicines?

If an error occurs in the administration or prescribing of medication who is responsible?

Prescribing of medicines is governed by statute, guidelines and policies. These set out when health professionals can administer drugs and what drugs can be administered.

There have been some very unsafe practices in the past, such as an unauthorised person prescribing medication then getting a doctor to write it up later. Prescribing errors occur for many reasons, including inadequate knowledge of the patient and their clinical condition, inadequate knowledge of the drug, calculation errors, incorrect dosage, omission of allergy status, inappropriate route of administration, no duration of treatment, drug name confusion, illegible handwriting and poor history taking. Factors such as fatigue and workload may contribute to the risk of error. There is a good reason why the prescribing and administering of medication is regulated; it provides a safe framework for practice.

If a patient is injured as a result of a prescription error or an error when administering, the health professional who made the error will be accountable. The patient may sue for compensation on the grounds of negligence. The health professional will be accountable to their employer and their professional body. Statutes and regulations apply to the prescribing and administering of medicines; a breach of these constitutes a criminal offence. There may also be criminal charges, for example, for an offence of assault and battery, if the medication has been administered without valid consent.

It is essential that the health professional is clear at all times which mechanism they are operating under, in order that they can comply with the legal, professional and clinical limits and requirements of that mechanism.

It is the responsibility of the health professional to be familiar with the laws and guidelines that relate to the prescribing and administering of medication.

EXAMPLE OF NON-COMPLIANCE

This case involved an elderly gentleman (the patient) who, for many years, had suffered intermittently from psoriasis and from time to time it would flare up. He was otherwise fit and mobile. On this occasion he had a flare up on the soles of his feet and a localised rash in the groin area.

The patient saw a consultant on a private basis who diagnosed psoriasis. As previous treatment of non-steroid anti-inflammatory cream had an adverse effect, arrangements were made for the patient to be admitted into hospital under the NHS to clear up the rash 'once and for all'.

On admission the consultant was away on a training course and would be away for the next seven days. There was no handover with this patient by the consultant and the private notes were not made available to the NHS hospital.

The patient was admitted by an SHO who wrote in the records, 'admitted with psoriasis'. The SHO also wrote in the clinical records 'allergy to penicillin', but did not record this allergy to penicillin on the drug chart or in the designated box on the front of the records.

For the first week the consultant was away on a course and did not see the patient. For the first four days the nursing staff applied non-steroid anti-inflammatory creams. On about day four, the rash had reddened and a blister had appeared in the groin area. A nurse had noticed this blister and telephoned several health professionals, including an SHO and registrar to seek advice as to how she should treat the patient. They could not assist so the nurse then telephoned the ward sister to ask for advice. She told the sister 'a blister has appeared, what do I do?' Without seeing the patient and over the telephone the ward sister prescribed Dermovate.

Dermovate is an extremely potent substance. It is a prescription-only medicine (for good reason – because of its potency). There were several problems at this point.

The ward sister did not have prescribing powers so was not suitably qualified to prescribe this medication.

There were contraindications for the use of Dermovate with this patient. For example, it should not be used in the folds of the skin, so it was inappropriate to use in the groin area. There were other contraindications: Dermovate is known to cause blistering.

For whatever reason – possibly because the nursing sister did not have prescribing powers or because she had given the advice over the telephone and did not have the records to hand – there was a failure by the nursing sister to write up the prescription on the drug chart.

The nurse made an entry in the nursing records that Dermovate was being applied.

The Dermovate exacerbated the patient's condition and localised blistering developed in the groin area. By day seven the rash had worsened and was by then quite a bullous rash.

On that day the consultant returned from his course. He is faced with a patient who has a bullous rash. He has the clinical records to hand but no nursing records and there is nothing recorded on the drug chart. The consultant is therefore ignorant of the fact that Dermovate is being applied and that this could be the cause of the rash.

On the basis of the clinical picture the consultant made a diagnosis of 'pemphigoid?' and made this entry in the record. Pemphigoid is a significant skin condition, but it is not immediately life threatening and it is easy to test for and diagnose then treat, or to rule it out.

However, no tests were carried out and no swabs or skin biopsies were taken. But on the basis of the clinical picture the consultant prescribed a high dose of steroid, 80 mg.

The following day the patient is catheterised. Over the following few days the catheter falls out. According to the records it had been pulled out by a nurse during bathing on at least two occasions, and then reinserted.

The patient's condition deteriorated, so the patient was prescribed penicillin! The patient developed an all-over rash – this, in a patient who is already suffering from a skin condition. The following day the error was realised and the penicillin was withdrawn.

However, the patient's condition continued to deteriorate. On day 12 the patient was reviewed by the consultant who considered that his condition was either 'pemphigoid or toxic epidermal necrolysis (TEN)' and made this entry in the records.

TEN is a life-threatening skin condition. It is a rare condition that affects the whole body where blisters occur and the epidermis peels off in large sheets. Widespread areas of erosion, including all mucous membranes (eyes, mouth, genitalia), occur within 24–72 hours, and the patient usually becomes gravely ill. Affected areas of skin often resemble second-degree burns. Death is caused by fluid and electrolyte imbalance and multi-organ sequelae (e.g. pneumonia, GI bleeding, glomerulonephritis, hepatitis, infection). A patient with TEN is usually treated as a burns patient, transferred to a burns unit, barrier nursed and so on.

However, this patient did not have these classic signs; he had a localised rash in the groin area. Neither was he treated as if he had TEN (i.e. transferred to burns unit, etc.).

TEN is a drug-induced condition and there are a handful of known drugs that cause this. But there was nothing they had given this patient, or at least there was nothing recorded on the drug chart, that could have caused TEN.

On the basis of this differential diagnosis of pemphigoid or TEN the consultant increased the steroid to 100 mg.

By day 14 the patient's condition had deteriorated further and the rash had not improved. The patient was reviewed by the consultant who considered that had it been TEN or pemphigoid then the steroid would have had some effect. So the plan was to 'withdraw steroid by tapering over the following four days'. The consultant made this entry in the records.

That day a nurse transposed this information from the clinical records into the nursing records as 'withdraw steroid'. Someone then drew a line through the steroid prescription on the drug chart, which resulted in the steroid being withdrawn abruptly.

The following day the patient had some coffee ground vomit. The patient went into shock and died the following day.

> This patient was admitted with nothing more than a localised rash of psoriasis, but within two weeks or so the patient had died as a result of prescribing errors and poor record keeping in relation to medication.

This case illustrates the dangers of prescribing outside of authorised powers to do so, poor records and poor communication. All health professionals involved would be accountable in this case in relation to prescribing.

➤ There was a failure by the SHO to record the allergy to penicillin in the designated box on the front of the records and on the drug chart, which resulted in the erroneous administering of penicillin.

➤ There was a failure by the nursing sister in prescribing Dermovate without prescribing powers and failing to record it on the drug chart, which resulted in the breakdown of communication.

➤ There was a failure by the consultant to have the nursing records to hand during the ward round, which resulted in a breakdown of communication.

➤ There was a failure by nursing staff incorrectly transposing information from the clinical records into the nursing records relating to the withdrawal of steroid and someone drawing a line through the prescription of steroid on the drug chart, which resulted in the abrupt withdrawal of the steroid causing the patient to go into shock.

The health professionals would be accountable to the deceased family who brought a claim for compensation. They will be accountable to the professional bodies. The nurse who prescribed outside her powers is committing a criminal offence.

General principles

The general principles regarding responsibility discussed in earlier chapters apply to prescribing and administering medication. For example, you cannot say 'I prescribed it because my boss told me to' or 'sorry, the prescription pad ran out'. This is not a defence and you will be accountable.

Medicinal products are regulated. The safest approach is to adopt the premise that it is unlawful to administer, prescribe or supply medicinal products unless it is done within one of the specific mechanisms permitting administration, prescription or supply. It is important to ensure that there is compliance with the conditions attached to the particular mechanism, such as under nurse prescribing, supplementary prescribing or a patient group directive, for example.

Legislation, policies and guidelines

The main legislation regarding the control, supply and administration of medicines is the:

➤ Medicines Act 1968
➤ Misuse of Drugs Act 1971, and statutory instruments including:
   — Misuse of Drugs Regulations 2001
   — Health Act 2006.

The regulation of medicines is undertaken by the Medicines and Healthcare Products Regulatory Authority (MHRA).[2]

The NMC has published guidelines for the administration of medicines which sets out a safe framework for practice.[3]

Local policies are also usually in place, which should be taken into account. Local policies must comply with the statutory framework.

As a consequence of the Shipman Inquiry and the use of controlled drugs in that case, a report was published and the law amended to reflect its recommendations. The Health Act 2006, sections 17–25 introduced new laws in relation to the supervision and management of the use of controlled drugs.[4] An accountable officer must now be appointed within each Trust to have a responsibility for the safe use and management of controlled drugs.

CLASSIFICATION OF MEDICINES

Medicinal drugs are classified into three categories to reflect their particular associated dangers and potential for misuse. The categories are Prescription-only medicines (POMs), Pharmacy medicines (P) and General sales list medicines (GSLs). Some Prescription-only medicines are further classified as Controlled drugs (CD).

The Medicines Act 1968,[5] which was prompted by the thalidomide experience, was introduced to bring together previous legislation and introduce new provisions for the control of medicines. It did not deal with dangerous drugs specifically, but many of its requirements apply to dangerous drugs. The Act specifies how each class should be dealt with.

➤ **Prescription-only medicines (POMs)** must only be sold or supplied on an appropriate practitioner's prescription and only be administered by an appropriate practitioner or on the direction of an appropriate practitioner. All controlled drugs are POMs unless they are below a certain strength as set out in Schedule 5 of the Misuse of Drugs Regulations 2001.[6]

➤ **Pharmacy medicines (P)** can only be sold or supplied from a registered pharmacy business and premises by or under the supervision of a pharmacist.

➤ **General sales list medicines (GSLs)** may be sold or supplied in a retail establishment other than a pharmacist, but only under the provisions of section 53 of the Medicines Act; that is, the place of sale is the premises where the business is carried out. It is a lockable premises and the medicine is in an unopened manufacturer's pack. None of the controlled drugs are GSLs.

➤ **Controlled drugs (CD)** are drugs that are considered 'dangerous'. They are regulated by the Misuse of Drugs Act 1971[7] and the Misuse of Drugs Regulations 2001.[8] It is unlawful to possess or supply a controlled drug (unless an exception or exemption applies). Under these provisions there are regulations regarding cultivation, production, supply, possession, prescription, marking, record-keeping, registers, provision of information, administration and destruction of controlled drugs. Breach of the regulations or any terms of a licence granted under the regulations is a criminal offence.

Responsible prescribing

Health professionals have an obligation to prescribe responsibly and in their patients' best interests, in accordance with the law and principles of professional standards.

It is a criminal offence to prescribe drugs other than to meet the identified needs of patients. Health professionals must make an appropriate assessment of the patient's condition, prescribe within their experience and competence and keep accurate records of the treatment.

Prescribing drugs is an integral aspect of many treatment plans, where the health professional has knowledge of the patient's health and medical history. It is important to have an understanding of the patient's current health and medication, including any relevant medical history, in order to prescribe drugs safely. If in doubt, the health professional should contact the patient's consultant, GP, general dental practitioner or other appropriate health professional, to clarify any queries.

Part of prescribing drugs responsibly means prescribing only where the health professional is able to form an objective view of the patient's health and clinical needs. Health professionals who prescribe drugs for themselves or those close to them may not be able to remain objective and risk overlooking serious problems, encouraging or tolerating addiction, or interfering with care or treatment provided by other healthcare professionals. Other than in emergencies, health professionals should not therefore prescribe drugs for themselves or for anyone with whom they have a close personal or emotional relationship.

MECHANISMS FOR PRESCRIBING, ADMINISTRATION AND SUPPLY
Who can prescribe and what can they prescribe?
An 'appropriate practitioner' can prescribe POMs.

Section 63 of the Health and Social Care Act 2001[9] enabled the government to extend prescribing responsibilities from doctors, dentists and vets to also include other health professionals, such as nurses and pharmacists. It also enabled the introduction of new types of prescribers including the concept of a supplementary prescriber.

What can be prescribed?
The NHS regulations define what drugs can be prescribed on the NHS.[10] The *British National Formulary* (BNF) contains a concise list of permissible drugs.[11]

Nurse independent prescribers
From 1 May 2006, nurse independent prescribers (formerly known as extended formulary nurse prescribers) who have completed the appropriate training can prescribe any licensed medicine for any clinical condition within their competence, including some controlled drugs.[12]

Nurse independent prescribers can prescribe any licensed medicine for any medical condition within their competence including some controlled drugs. They can prescribe a licensed medicine 'off-label' or 'off-licence'; however, they must take full clinical and professional responsibility for their prescribing and should only prescribe 'off-label' where it is best practice to do so. They cannot prescribe an unlicensed medicine. However, nurse independent prescribers who are also supplementary prescribers can still prescribe them as part of a supplementary prescribing arrangement, if the doctor agrees within a clinical management plan.

Community practitioner nurse prescribers

Community practitioner nurse prescribers, such as district nurses, health visitors, general practice nurses and school nurses, can only prescribe dressings, appliances and licensed medicines from the Nurse Prescribers' Formulary for Community Practitioners.[13]

They do not undertake the same depth of prescribing training as nurse independent prescribers and should not prescribe 'off-label' apart from very limited exceptions. The community nurse prescriber must be familiar with products that may be exceptionally prescribed off-label.

The community practitioner nurse prescribers that prescribe off-label must be clear that they accept clinical and medico-legal responsibility for prescribing that medicine. Community practitioner nurse prescribers should only prescribe the permitted 'off-label' medication within their own competence and where they are clear of the correct diagnosis.

Pharmacist independent prescriber

From 1 May 2006 the qualified pharmacist independent prescriber type was introduced.[14] Once qualified, pharmacist independent prescribers can prescribe any licensed medicine for any clinical condition within their professional and clinical competence, except for controlled drugs.

INDEPENDENT AND SUPPLEMENTARY PRESCRIBERS

Independent prescribers

The independent prescriber should be the clinician responsible for the individual's care at the time that supplementary prescribing is to start.

Responsibility

Independent prescribing means that the prescriber takes responsibility for:
➤ clinical assessment of the patient
➤ establishing a diagnosis
➤ establishing clinical management required
➤ prescribing.

The independent prescriber must:
➤ make a diagnosis
➤ make decisions about the clinical management required

➤ make decisions about prescribing
➤ make decisions about the continuing care of the patient
➤ make decisions about patient review.

The independent prescriber must reach agreement with the supplementary prescriber about the limits of their responsibility for prescribing and review and sharing the patient's records with the supplementary prescriber.

Supplementary prescribing

Section 63 of the Health and Social Care Act 2001[15] enabled the government to extend prescribing responsibilities and introduced the concept of the supplementary prescriber. They include pharmacists, chiropodists, podiatrists, physiotherapists, optometrists and radiographers who are qualified, registered and have undergone specialist training.

Supplementary prescribing is 'a voluntary partnership between an independent prescriber and a supplementary prescriber to implement an agreed patient specific clinical management plan with the patient's agreement'.[16]

What are the parameters?

Supplementary prescribers may prescribe any NHS medicine provided it is in partnership with an independent prescriber who gives the initial diagnosis and starts the treatment. The supplementary prescriber then monitors the patient and prescribes further supplies of medication when necessary. Prescription of any medicine, including controlled drugs and unlicensed medicines are permitted.

Responsibility

Supplementary prescribing involves both the independent prescriber and dependant (supplementary) prescriber. The independent prescriber would be responsible for the assessment of patients with undiagnosed conditions and for decisions about the clinical management required, including prescribing. The dependant (supplementary) prescriber would be responsible for the continuing care of patients who have been clinically assessed by an independent prescriber.

Supplementary prescribers may also be involved in continuing established treatments by issuing repeat prescriptions, with authority to adjust the dose or dosage form according to the patient's needs. There should be provision for regular review by the assessing clinician.

The supplementary prescriber:

➤ must be competent to prescribe
➤ may prescribe for the full range of medical conditions providing it is in accordance with the clinical management plan
➤ should pass prescribing responsibility back to the independent prescriber if the clinical reviews are not carried out within the specified intervals or if they feel that the patient's condition no longer falls within their competence
➤ must record prescribing and monitoring activity contemporaneously in the shared patient record.

For the supplementary prescriber there is no legal restriction on the clinical conditions that they may treat.

There must be access to common patient records and there must be a clinical management plan in place before treatment can begin.

The high cost of litigation is largely as a result of breakdowns in communication.

The clinical management plan is a key document for the communication of patient care; it is the cornerstone of supplementary prescribing.

A nurse independent prescriber may also operate under the mechanism of a supplementary prescriber notwithstanding their own prescribing powers.

PATIENT GROUP DIRECTIVES

A patient group directive (PGD) is a written instruction for the supply or administration of medicines to groups of patients who may not be individually identified before presentation for treatment. PGDs allow the supply and administration of specified medicines to patients who fall into a group defined in the PGD; using a PGD is not a form of prescribing.

Patient group directives can only be used by registered nurses, midwives, health visitors, paramedics, chiropodists, dieticians, occupational therapists, optometrists, orthoptists, physiotherapists, pharmacists, prosthetists, radiographers, and speech and language therapists who are named in a list held by their organisation.

Unlike nurse and pharmacist prescribing, healthcare professionals entitled to work with a PGD require no additional formal qualification. However, for a PGD to be valid, certain criteria must be met both in terms of the patient group that the PGD can be used for, and in how the PGD itself is drawn up.

Organisations also have a responsibility to ensure that only fully competent, trained healthcare professionals use PGDs.

Although patient group directives have their place, the preferred way for patients to receive medicines is for an appropriately qualified healthcare professional to prescribe for an individual patient on a one-to-one basis.

UNLICENSED MEDICINES

In the UK, no medicine for human use may be placed upon the market without first being granted a product license by the licensing authority (the Medicines Control Agency). In considering a licence application the licensing authority gives particular consideration to the safety, efficacy, and quality of the product. This is put in place to protect the public, and ensures that the medicines on the market are of the appropriate quality. However, an exemption exists to allow prescribers to use unlicensed medicines to meet the special needs of a patient.

Trusts should have a policy in place to enable the management to monitor and manage the risks associated with the use of unlicensed medicines.

Only doctors, dentists and vets can prescribe unlicensed medicines. Nurse independent prescribers cannot prescribe unlicensed medicines.

Types of unlicensed medicines and unlicensed use

Types of unlicensed medicines fall into four broad categories.

1 Unlicensed medicines derived from licensed materials; for example, liquid preparations for those unable to swallow, creams and ointments not commercially available. These may be prepared under a 'specials' manufacturing licence by a commercial supplier, or for infrequently used products, by the hospital pharmacy under a Medicines Act exemption.
2 Products unrelated to licensed medicines and for which a licence has yet to be granted.
3 Products which have had their product licence abandoned, revoked, suspended or not renewed.
4 Drugs in clinical trials.

The use of a medicine is also unlicensed if it is used outside of the indication stated in its product licence.

Whilst prescribers will generally prescribe licensed products, the law allows them to prescribe unlicensed medicines, or use licensed products for an unlicensed purpose for the special needs of their particular patient. Issues arise in relation to advice given to the patient and also in respect of the quality of the product.

Nurse prescribers can prescribe 'off licence' but remember they cannot prescribe unlicensed medicines.

The health professional who prescribes unlicensed medicines will be accountable.

The health professional must be aware of the licensing status when prescribing unlicensed medicine or a licensed medicine outside of its product licence. It is also important that when obtaining consent for treatment, the prescriber should, where possible, inform the patient of the medicine's licensed status in terms they can understand and that for an unlicensed medicine its effects will be less understood than for those of a licensed medicine.

It is recognised that the prescriber may not know the licensed status of the drug to be supplied to the patient, and therefore the pharmacist has a role in identifying the status of these products and should bring this to the attention of the prescriber.

PRESCRIPTIONS

A prescription-only medicine should not be sold or supplied in accordance with a prescription unless:

➤ it is signed in ink with the name of the appropriate practitioner
➤ it is written in ink or otherwise so as to be indelible if it is for a controlled drug
➤ it has the following particulars:
  — the address of the appropriate practitioner
  — the appropriate date (date signed or specified, before which it should not be prescribed)
  — an indication whether the appropriate practitioner is a doctor or dentist etc.
  — the name, address and age of the person for whom the treatment is given if under 12 years old
  — it is not to be dispensed after six months from appropriate date unless it is a repeatable prescription.

There is a prescribed form for prescriptions appropriate to the health professional issuing it.

ADMINISTERING DRUGS

Administration

Regulations in relation to the administering of drugs include parenteral administration, which may only be administered as follows:

➤ self-administered, or

➤ administered by a doctor or dentist, or

➤ administered by an independent nurse prescriber or a supplementary prescriber subject to limitations, or

➤ anyone acting in accordance with a patient specific direction (PSD) of a doctor or an independent nurse prescriber or supplementary prescriber (subject to limitations).

Covert administration of medicine

It is the basic legal principle that when treating a patient, including administering medication, consent to such treatment is obtained from them. Covert administration of medicines will never apply to patients who have capacity, even if it were life saving. However, there may be occasions where the patient lacks capacity to consent to their treatment. Covert administration may only be justified where the patient lacks capacity and it is in the best interest of the patient to administer it in this way.

In respect of covert administration health professionals should consider the following:

➤ there must be clear evidence that the patient lacks capacity

➤ the best interest of the patient must be considered at all times

➤ the decision to administer covertly should not be considered routine and should be a contingency measure

➤ the decisions should be reached after assessing the care needs of the patient

➤ it should be patient-specific to avoid routine covert administration

➤ there should be broad and open discussion among the multidisciplinary team and supporters of the client such as carers, relatives and advocates, with agreement that this approach is required

➤ the method should be agreed with the pharmacist

➤ the decision, action taken and parties involved should be well documented

➤ it should be reviewed at regular intervals

➤ attempts to encourage the patient to take medication should be made regularly

➤ there should be written local policy having regard to professional guidelines.

ACCESS, CONTROL AND DESTRUCTION

A list of controlled drugs can be found in the *BNF*.[17] The health professional must be familiar with the procedure for access to controlled drugs stock, their destruction and record keeping. Health professionals should always have easy access to a copy of the *BNF*.

All health professionals should go through a checklist before a drug is administered to a patient. The health professional must ensure they fulfil their duties according to the approved standards of practice expected. If something goes wrong the health professional will be accountable. If a patient is harmed as a result of a drug error the health professional will be accountable to the patient, who may sue for negligence; to their professional body; to their employer; and to the criminal courts. (*See* checklist in Figure 2.1.)

RESPONSIBILITY

It is very important that health professionals prescribe within their powers. It is illegal to prescribe outside their powers and they will be accountable.

The health professional must ensure that there is no conflict of interest when prescribing. Prescribing powers must not be used for the promotion of commercial products or services. A gift from a pharmaceutical company may be seen as promotion of commercial products or services.

A nurse prescriber can only prescribe medicine for a patient he or she has assessed for care.

Another nurse prescriber may issue a repeat prescription in the absence of the original nurse prescriber. Accountability rests with the nurse who issued that prescription. Nurse prescribers may give patient-specific directions to another person but must be satisfied that the person is competent to administer the medicine.

Nurse prescribers must ensure that the patient is aware of the scope and limits of nurse prescribing.

Vicarious liability

If a nurse prescribes outside their powers they will be accountable. The NMC is making it clear that such action is in breach of the code of conduct and that employers may not stand by them if a claim for compensation for negligence is made.

It is recommended that health professionals take out professional indemnity insurance in the event that the employer considers that they have been acting outside their powers of prescribing and the employer is therefore not vicariously liable for their actions.

If a health professional does not have professional indemnity insurance they must inform the patient beforehand.

The health professional must also remember that simply because they have insurance in place or their employer accepts vicarious liability the health professional is still accountable in the areas discussed in Chapter 2.

Acting in an emergency

Prescription-only medicines may be administered without the direction of the doctor, where the situation is an emergency for the purpose of saving the patient's life; for example, a parent or teacher who needs to administer adrenalin when a child has suffered anaphylactic shock.

Conflict with the prescriber

A health professional may consider that the prescription written up by a doctor is inappropriate. What should the health professional do in the circumstances? Who is accountable if the prescribed medication causes harm to the patient?

EXAMPLE OF CONFLICT WITH THE PRESCRIBER

Susan is a geriatric nurse with three years experience. An elderly patient is admitted with suspected meningitis. The doctor on call writes a prescription for a high dose of antibiotics. Susan queries the dose with the doctor who is furious at her questioning. The doctor insists that Susan administers the antibiotic in the prescribed dose and timings. As Susan has only three years experience in geriatrics she is uncertain how to deal with the situation. She knows that the patient is seriously ill and that the high dose may be justified in the circumstances and that the patient required urgent treatment.

What is the responsibility of Susan?

In these circumstances, Susan will be accountable for administering the drugs. She must check the prescription in all circumstances, even where considerable pressure is placed upon her.

Only in a dire emergency may she be able to rely on the fact that the doctor ordered her to give the drug and not have the opportunity to question the dosage because of the seriousness of the patient's condition and the urgent need for treatment.

Susan should inform her manager of her concerns and should ask a more senior doctor to confirm that the medication, dosage, timing and route are correct. Ideally she should also check with the pharmacist. She should inform the doctor that she is refusing to administer the drug and the doctor has the option of either administering it himself or rethinking his position.

Susan, however, risks disciplinary action for her refusal, if such refusal to administer was deemed unreasonable.

Strict product liability (liability without fault)

Strict product liability means that if a patient can demonstrate that he has suffered injury whilst undergoing a course of treatment and the medicine was defective, then he can bring an action for damages against the manufacturer of the product without needing to prove negligence. This applies to all medicinal products. In the case of a licensed product, the liability would rest with the product licence holder. However, because an unlicensed medicine cannot be offered for sale, but rather is procured or commissioned by a purchaser, the purchaser retains responsibility for the quality of the product; the manufacturer is considered to be a subcontractor acting under directions. This has the effect that if a hospital provides medicine that is defective, they will nevertheless be responsible to the patient for harm caused. However, the Trust may then look to the manufacturer to try to recoup their loss.

A further consideration that needs to be taken into account is the extent of the exemption that allows the use of unlicensed medicines. The current interpretation is that the exemption is intended to cover exceptional circumstances where no suitable licensed product is available. This means that where a licensed product is available then that product should be used.

The degree of risk encountered will vary depending upon the circumstances in which a medicine is used. A medicine that has had its licensed revoked or suspended is likely to provide a greater risk than one that is unlicensed simply because a suitable formulation is not available.

MEDICATION AND LACK OF RESOURCES

As discussed in the chapter on resources, the law recognises reasonable management of resources. A patient cannot demand a course of treatment. As long as a suitable medication is prescribed it does not have to be the best or most expensive just because the patient has asked for it.

CASE

Herceptin
A woman who was refused Herceptin by her local Trust took her case to the court. A doctor had identified that her condition was such that she required the drug. They said that the Trust could not refuse to give her the drug on the grounds of cost alone.

If the health professional has assessed the patient as requiring certain medication then a failure to provide it may be a breach of duty. The media attention in relation to the breast cancer drug, Herceptin, is an example of this.

RECORD KEEPING AND MEDICINES

Record keeping

The same best practice principles apply to record keeping in respect of medication as to any other health records.

The Misuse of Drugs Regulations[18] enables all details on prescriptions for controlled drugs to be computer generated, except for a signature.

Illegible writing

All records should be written clearly and legibly.

Health professionals should take care to ensure that their entries can be read by others. If a mistake is made because your writing is illegible you will be accountable. If you cannot read the writing of another health professional or if there is any doubt about the drug prescribed, you should take steps to find out what it reads. The health professional should not administer it unless they have checked it with the doctor who has prescribed it. If the health professional does not do this and they act on illegible records, they, as well as the writer, will be accountable.

Calculation errors

Many prescribing errors have occurred due to calculation errors. These have often occurred where the entries are illegible, in particular in relation to decimal points being incorrectly placed, for example, where 5 mL has been administered instead of 0.5 mL.

> *The Times* in October 2000 reported that a baby in the neonatal unit died where a decimal point in a drug prescription was entered in the wrong place.[19]

Health professionals will be accountable if a failure to appropriately calculate the medication dose causes harm to the patient.

Intravenous

Since 1975 at least 13 patients in the UK have died or been paralysed as a result of being injected by the anti-cancer drug vincristine.

CASE

Incorrect administration

In 2001, a teenager died as a result of a junior doctor administering vincristine, which was accidentally injected into his spine instead of a vein.[20] The doctor pleaded guilty to the manslaughter.

As mentioned previously in Chapter 11, in the section on system failures, it was recommended that a spinal syringe should be designed so it cannot physically be joined into an ampoule containing a drug that should not be given spinally.

Guidelines have been published by the Department of Health in 2008 on the safety of administering intrathecal chemotherapy.[21]

Telephone advice

The dangers of advising over the telephone are highlighted in the case study at the beginning of this chapter. Giving instructions by telephone to a health professional to administer a previously unprescribed substance is not acceptable.

Where medication has been previously prescribed and the prescriber is unable to issue a new prescription with changes to the dose considered to be necessary, then written instructions should be given, by e-mail, fax or text message.[22]

CONSENT

When prescribing and administering medication it is important for the health professionals to keep in mind the issues of consent.

The health professional must provide sufficient information to the patient regarding the medication, such as risks. Remember to consider the ingredients of the medication, which may cause an allergic reaction, or ingredients that may cause offence to the patient, such as animal products that may not be suitable for vegetarians or those of certain faiths.

Consent is a complex area and is not within the ambit of this book. Health professionals should be familiar with the issues of consent when prescribing or administering medication.

CHECKLIST FOR PRESCRIBING

Check	Clarify the issues
Correct patient	Ensure that you have the correct patient. You should check the records and be sure there can be no mix up. Health professionals should have particular regard to issues of family members who may have the same name, or where names are common.
Consent	Does the patient have capacity to consent?
	Are they suffering from a mental illness or mental handicap?
	Is the patient an adult or child?
	Has the patient received all of the relevant information?
	Have you taken into account whether the patient has a pre-existing condition?
	Are there any contraindications?
	Has the patient been informed of the risks?
The drug	Has the drug been checked as correct?
	Have the side-effects been considered?
	Is the timing correct?
	Are there any special precautions?
	Are there any contraindications?
	Ensure the drug is in date and has not expired.
The dose	Has the correct dose been checked?
	Consider the type of patient.
	Consider the physique of the patient.
	Consider if there is an allergy and the frequency of the allergy.
Method and site of administration	Oral or injection.
	Injection: intramuscular or intravenous?
	Skin (external application).
	Injection site.
Procedure	Ensure correct procedure is followed.
	Does the administrator have the competence, skill and training?
	Has the administration been delegated appropriately?
	Is it the correct gauge of needle?
	Is the equipment safe?
	Is the procedure sterile?
Record keeping	Have you ensured a good record is made in the appropriate sections in the records of the drug, the dose, the time the drug is administered and the method of administration?

REFERENCES

1 Health and Social Care Act 2001 section 63.

2 www.mhra.gov.uk

3 Nursing and Midwifery Council. *Standards for Medicine Management*. London: NMC; 2008. Available at: www.nmc-uk.org/aDisplayDocument.aspx?documentID=4676 (accessed 30 March 2009).

4 Health Act 2006.

5 Medicines Act 1968.

6 Misuse of Drugs Regulations 2001 schedule 5.

7 Misuse of Drugs Act 1971.

8 Misuse of Drugs Regulations 2001.

9 Health and Social Care Act, op. cit.

10 National Health Service (General Medical Services Contracts) Regulations 2004.

11 *BNF* No 57, Annex: Dental Practitioners' Formulary, Annex: Nurse Prescribers' Formulary, Annex: Non-medical prescribing.

12 Department of Health. *Nurse Independent Prescribing*. London: DoH; 2006. Available at: www.dh.gov.uk/en/Healthcare/Medicinespharmacyandindustry/Prescriptions/TheNon-MedicalPrescribingProgramme/Nurseprescribing/index.htm (accessed 30 March 2009).

13 *BNF* No 57, Annex: Nurse Prescribers' Formulary.

14 Department of Health. *Improving Patients' Access to Medicines: A guide to implementing nurse and pharmacist independent prescribing within the NHS in England*. London: DoH; 2006. Available at: www.dh.gov.uk/en/publicationsandstatistics/publications/publicationspolicyandguidance/dh_4133743 (accessed 20 April 2009).

15 Health and Social Care Act, op. cit.

16 Department of Health. *About Supplementary Prescribing*. London: DoH; 2007. Available at: www.dh.gov.uk/en/Healthcare/Medicinespharmacyandindustry/Prescriptions/TheNonMedicalPrescribingProgramme/Supplementaryprescribing/DH_4123025 (accessed 20 April 2009).

17 *BNF*, op. cit.

18 Misuse of Drugs Regulations 2001, op. cit.

19 Hurst G. Baby dies after one decimal point drug dose error. *The Times*. 11 Oct 2000.

20 Laville S, Hall C, McIlroy AJ. Vincristine. *The Telegraph*. 19 June 2001.

21 Department of Health. *Updated National Guidance on the Safe Administration of Intrathecal Chemotherapy*. HSC 2008/001. London: DoH; 2008. Available at: www.dh.gov.uk/en/Publicationsandstatistics/Lettersandcirculars/Healthservicecirculars/DH_086870 (accessed 20 April 2009).

22 Nursing and Midwifery Council. *Standards for Medicines Management*. London: NMC; 2008. Available at: www.nmc-uk.org/aDisplayDocument.aspx?documentID=4585 (accessed 20 April 2009).

Glossary

Accountability	Someone who is accountable is completely responsible for what they do and must be able to give a satisfactory reason for it.
Act of Parliament	A document that sets out legal rules.
Actus reus	'The guilty act', the physical act of a crime. An essential element of a crime that must be proved to secure a conviction.
Adversarial	Approach in court involving or characterised by conflict or opposition.
Assault and battery	Assault is an intentional or reckless act that causes someone to expect to be subjected to immediate physical harm. Battery is an intentional or negligent application of physical force.
Balance of probability	Establishing the facts to the satisfaction of the court. The standard of proof in civil proceedings is on the balance of probabilities.
Bar	The profession of barrister.
Barrister	A lawyer qualified to present the case in court.
Breach of duty	An act of breaking a law. Where there is a duty of care and that duty has not been met. Negligence is also referred to as a breach of the duty of care.
Beyond reasonable doubt	Establishing the facts to the satisfaction of the court. The standard of proof in criminal proceedings is beyond reasonable doubt.

Civil law	The legal system which relates to personal matters, such as marriage and property, rather than criminal matters.
Claimant	A person who brings a claim (sues) for something which they believe they have a right to.
Cohorted	Patients with the same infection can be nursed together (cohorted) in one room, rather than in individual rooms (isolation).
Common law	The legal system developed over a period of time from old customs and court decisions, rather than laws made in parliament.
Compensation	Monetary payment to compensate for loss or damage. Also referred to as damages.
Contemporaneously	Happening or existing at the same period of time.
Criminal law	The legal system which relates to punishing people who break the law.
Contraindication	A sign that someone should not continue with a particular medicine or treatment because it is or might be harmful.
Coroner	A person appointed to hold an inquiry (inquest) into a death that occurred in unexpected or unusual circumstances.
Crown Prosecution Service	CPS is responsible for prosecuting people in England and Wales charged with a criminal offence.
Cardiotochograph	CTG is an electronic record in the form of a graph used to monitor the fetal heart rate during pregnancy.
Counsel	Another name for a barrister.
Damages	Monetary payment to compensate for loss or damage. Also referred to as compensation.
Declaration	A ruling by the court setting out the legal situation.
Defendant	A person in a law case who is accused of having done something unlawful.
Dermatologist	A doctor who studies and treats skin diseases.
Dermovate	Medication containing corticosteroid which is used to decrease inflammation in the skin.

Disclosure	Documents made available to another party or the court.
Duty of care	The legal obligation.
Ectopic pregnancy	An ectopic pregnancy occurs when the fertilised egg attaches itself outside the cavity of the uterus (womb). The majority of ectopic pregnancies are found in the fallopian tubes.
Employment tribunal	A legal process to hear and rule on disputes between employers and employees.
Fraud	A false representation by a statement or conduct in order to gain a material advantage.
General Dental Council	GDC is the professional body for dentists.
General Medical Council	GMC is the professional body for doctors.
House of Lords	The highest appeal court in England and Wales.
Health Professions Council	HPC is the professional body for allied health professionals.
Inquest	A court process to discover the cause of someone's death.
Intrapartum	In the womb, referring to when the foetus is still in the womb.
Intrathecally	Administration of drugs by injection into the spinal fluid
Law reports	Reports of cases decided by the courts.
Lawyer	A person who practises or studies law such as a solicitor or a barrister.
Liability/liable	Responsible for the wrongdoing or harm in civil proceedings.
Lipoma	A fatty growth often found on the breast which causes a lump that changes the shape of the breast. It requires no treatment.
Litigation	The process of taking a case to a law court so that an official decision can be made.
Magistrate	Justice of the Peace, a civil officer who administers the law in the magistrates court.
Metastised	Spreading of cancer from the primary source.

Mens rea	'The guilty mind', the mental element of a crime. An essential element of a crime that must be proved to secure a conviction.
Negligence	Failure to do something or doing something that a reasonable person would not do. Breach of the duty of care is also referred to as negligence.
National Health Service Litigation Authority	NHSLA is a Special Health Authority (part of the NHS), responsible for handling negligence claims made against NHS bodies in England.
National Institute for Health and Clinical Excellence	NICE is an independent organisation responsible for providing national guidance on promoting good health and preventing and treating ill health.
Nursing and Midwifery Council	NMC is the professional body for nurses and midwives.
No win no fee	An agreement where legal costs will not be recovered by a solicitor if a claim for compensation is unsuccessful.
Pemphigoid	An autoimmune disease that causes blistering of the skin.
Patient Group Directive	PGD is written instructions for the supply or administration of named medicines to specific groups of patients who may not be individually identified before presenting for treatment.
Postnatal	After the baby has been born.
Pre-action protocol	Rules that provide guidance on action to be taken before legal proceedings commence.
Primary Care Trust	PCTs provide primary care services which are the first point of call for a patient. For example, GP practices, pharmacists, dentists and opticians. The PCTs also manage community services such as district nursing, community hospitals and clinics.
Psoriasis	A chronic, recurring skin disease that causes one or more raised, red patches that have silvery scales and a distinct border between the patch and normal skin.
Recklessness	Doing something dangerous and not caring about the risks and the possible results.

Rigor	Sudden attack of severe shivering with feeling of coldness indicating a sudden worsening of a fever.
Solicitor	A lawyer qualified to manage legal cases, give legal advice to clients, and represent clients in lower courts.
Standard of proof	Establishing the facts to the satisfaction of the court. The standard of proof in criminal proceedings is beyond reasonable doubt. The standard of proof in civil proceedings is on the balance of probabilities.
Statute	Act of parliament.
Strict liability	Liability for the criminal act where the mental element does not have to be proved.
Sue	Take legal action against a person or organization by making a legal claim for money because of some harm that they have caused.
Toxic epidermal necrolysis	TEN is a life-threatening skin disease that causes a rash, skin peeling, and sores on the mucous membranes.
Theft	Dishonestly taking property belonging to another.
Tort	A wrongful act or omission for which compensation can be claimed.
Trespass	A wrongful direct interference with another person or with their property.
Vicarious liability	Legal liability imposed on one person or organisation for the torts or crimes of another. Usually, an employer is vicariously liable for its employees.
Witness	A person who gives evidence of what they saw, did or heard.

Index